The American
Dietetic
Association
Guide to

Women's Nutrition

for Healthy Living

Most Perigee Books are available at special quantity discounts for
bulk purchases for sales promotions, premiums, fund-raising or educational use. Special books, or book excerpts, can also be created
to fit specific needs.

For details write: Special Markets, The Berkley Publishing Group,
200 Madison Avenue, New York, New York 10016.

The
American
Dietetic
Association
Guide to

Women's Nutrition
for Healthy Living

Susan Calvert Finn, Ph.D., R.D., F.A.D.A.
with Jane Grant Tougas

Foreword by Bernadine Healy, M.D.

A PERIGEE BOOK

A Perigee Book
Published by The Berkley Publishing Group
A member of Penguin Putnam Inc.
200 Madison Avenue
New York, NY 10016

Copyright © 1997 by The American Dietetic Association
Book design by Irving Perkins Associates, Inc.
Cover design by Elizabeth Sheehan

First edition: October 1997

Published simultaneously in Canada.

The Putnam Berkley World Wide Web side address is http://www.berkley.com

Library of Congress Cataloging-in-Publication Data

Finn, Susan Calvert.
    The American Dietetic Association guide to women's nutrition for healthy living / Susan Calvert Finn ; with a foreword by Bernadine P. Healy.
        p.   cm.
    "A Perigee book"
    ISBN 0-399-52342-1
    1. Women—Nutrition.   I. Title.
    RA778.F48   1997
    613.2'082—DC21   97-9772
                                                                         CIP

Printed in the United States of America

10   9   8   7   6   5   4   3   2

Notice: The information in this book is true and complete to the best of our knowledge. In no way is this book intended to replace, countermand or conflict with the advice given to you by your doctor. The information in this book is general and is offered with no guarantees on the part of the authors or the publisher. The authors and publisher disclaim all liability in connection with the use of this book.

*This book is dedicated
to the healing spirit in all women*

Contents

Foreword

$\mathcal{A}$lmost a decade ago, I delivered the keynote address at The American Dietetic Association (ADA) annual meeting. A cardiologist by training, I was at the time president of the American Heart Association (AHA) and the first AHA president invited to be an ADA keynoter.

I spoke about the shared mission of the American Heart Association and The American Dietetic Association in promoting low-fat, low-cholesterol diets for heart health. At the time, the AHA had initiated a nationwide campaign against heart disease in women. As this campaign took root, my faith in women as leaders on the frontiers of health proved to be well placed. Thousands of AHA volunteers, most of them women, rallied to the cause.

I concluded that ADA speech with a reminder of the important role of women in our fight against heart disease, noting the high representation of women in fields that influence lifestyle—like dietetics, pediatrics, nursing, teaching and parenting. Now, looking back over the last ten years, it is clear that The American Dietetic Association and I have followed parallel paths in promoting the role of nutrition in women's health—and the role of women in society's health.

I believe nutrition is the single most important factor in the health and well-being of women at any stage of life. Indeed, this belief is a central premise of my recent book, *A New Prescription for Women's Health: Getting the Best Medical Care in a Man's World* (Penguin, 1996). Among the ten women's health topics I explored in this book, nutrition was number one. The American Dietetic Association's Nutrition and Health Campaign for Women also places nutrition at the top of the list for the prevention and treatment of diseases to which women are vulnerable. The ADA shares my feeling that it is critical to help women realize nutrition is an important aspect of health risk we can control. We can't change our age or heredity, but we can change what we eat, and by doing so we can make significant changes in our well-being. So we must learn more about how diet affects women's health. (And we must use what we learn; a good first step would be requiring medical schools to include nutrition in their curricula.)

As director of the National Institutes of Health (NIH), I gained an insider's perspective on the weakness of the research infrastructure underpinning women's health. To strengthen this research base, we launched the Women's Health Initiative, a multiyear, $625-million study of the diseases that affect women. The Initiative is exploring causes, risk factors, prevention and treatment for diseases such as breast cancer, heart disease and osteoporosis—not just as single entities but in relation to one another. In this context of total health, researchers are also studying the effects of behavioral factors such as nutrition and exercise on these diseases. The ADA shares this commitment to research and has funded studies targeting specific nutrition concerns in women's health.

With the NIH Women's Health Initiative under way and the ADA's Nutrition and Health Campaign for Women in full swing, I believe we are wonderfully positioned for a great expansion of knowledge in women's health. Dr. Susan Finn's book is a valuable contribution to this effort.

Susan Calvert Finn, Ph.D., R.D., F.A.D.A., is a former president of The American Dietetic Association and my colleague in the pursuit of better health and health care for women. She is a central architect of the ADA's Nutrition and Health Campaign for Women and serves as its chief spokesperson. Under her insightful leadership, the ADA has worked with other key nutrition and health organizations to shape the national agenda on women's health.

Dr. Finn believes, as I do, that it's time to shift our perspective away from avoiding nutritional deficiencies and toward understanding how nutrition helps prevent disease. To do this, we must—like the researchers—place nutrition in the context of total health, and that's exactly what Dr. Finn does in this book. She clearly delineates the issues and offers sound, practical nutritional advice—all with a healthy dose of inspiration.

You will find Dr. Finn's approach to nutrition very accessible and her enthusiasm contagious. I hope you come away from this book sharing our commitment to improving women's nutritional health—starting with your own.

—Bernadine Healy, M.D.
Former Director,
National Institutes of Health;
Dean, College of Medicine,
The Ohio State University
Columbus, Ohio

Preface

*W*hen The American Dietetic Association (ADA) asked me to chair its Nutrition and Health Campaign for Women, I eagerly embraced the opportunity. I knew that no group was better suited to helping women take charge of their nutritional health than the 70,000-member American Dietetic Association, the world's largest group of food and nutrition professionals.

Over the past three years, ADA has worked closely with other nutrition organizations, women's health advocates and policy makers to ensure that women's health issues remain high on the national agenda. This effort continues today as does our initiative to educate the media not only on women's health issues but also on how to interpret and responsibly report research findings. ADA has funded six research projects that will contribute valuable data to the ongoing exploration of women's unique health and nutritional needs.

This book, *The American Dietetic Association Guide to Women's Nutrition for Healthy Living,* is another component of ADA's Nutrition and Health Campaign for Women. Impetus for this project came from a Gallup survey of 1,000 women commissioned by ADA and Weight Watchers International. In that study, nearly 80 percent of respondents expressed concern about the effect of food choices on their future health. The same survey, however, revealed that, despite their knowledge of the importance of good nutrition, less than a third of respondents described their diet as very healthy.

The media has been scurrying to bridge what I call this "health-action" gap. The major news weeklies have devoted cover stories to dietary fat, obesity and obesity drugs. Food manufacturers are jumping into the fray as well. While watching prime time television one night I saw commercials extolling the cancer-fighting benefits of orange juice, the folic acid content of orange juice, the vitamins in bread, the calcium in yogurt, low-fat cake mix and low-fat fast food sandwiches—all in the space of one thirty-minute program.

Although much of this information is timely, accurate and potentially useful, it is nonetheless fragmented. Bombarded with all of this data, you, like many women, may ask: "What am I supposed to *do*?"

The American Dietetic Association Guide to Women's Nutrition for Healthy Living answers that question by giving you the tools you need to act—and act now. I have focused on contemporary nutrition issues and dilemmas, while helping you build solid, practical personal nutrition management skills. By emphasizing the importance of nutritional health over the course of a woman's lifetime, I hope to bring daughters, mothers, granddaughters and grandmothers together in a mutual effort to improve their health by making good nutrition part of their lifestyles.

Throughout the book, I have pointed out times when it is wise to discuss your individual needs or concerns with your physician or with a nutrition professional. Physicians are becoming more knowledgeable about the role of nutrition in health, especially as our health care system becomes more prevention oriented. Unfortunately, however, nutrition in general and the nutritional concerns of women in particular are still not well integrated into medical school curricula.

You may want to ask your physician for a referral to a registered dietitian (R.D.), who can review your nutritional health history and help you frame a plan for the future. You can be assured that a registered dietitian has completed a rigorous educational program and internship. R.D.s must also pursue regular continuing education in order to keep their certification. Some states also license registered dietitians to further protect consumers from unqualified practitioners. If you need help finding a registered dietitian in your area, call ADA's Nutrition Hot Line, (800) 366-1655.

I would like to thank The American Dietetic Association for involving me in this important initiative to improve the nutritional health of women. Special appreciation goes to my campaign cochair, Deborah McBride, ADA's director of publications, and to my writing partner, Jane Grant Tougas. I also want to acknowledge and thank my editor, Sheila Curry; my literary agent, Lynn Rosen; and the four nutrition professionals who reviewed the text for accuracy: Ann M. Coulston, M.S., R.D., F.A.D.A., research dietitian, Stanford University Medical Center; Jean H. Hankin, Ph.D., R.D., nutrition researcher and professor, Cancer Research Center, University of Hawaii; Penny Kris-Etherton, Ph.D., R.D., distinguished professor of nutrition, Pennsylvania State University; and Rosemary Riley, Ph.D., of Ross Laboratories.

I am also grateful to my employer, Abbott Laboratories, especially to Ross Products Division president Tom McNally and to Abbott chairman Duane L. Burnham for their continuing commitment to women's health. Thanks also to my staff and my professional colleagues for encouraging me and helping me to pursue my passion for women's health. And I want to thank my family as well, especially my husband, Jim, who cares about women's health as much as I do.

And for you, the reader, I hope this book will be your first step toward a long and healthy journey through life.

Introduction

*W*hether you are a senior, a baby boomer or a member of the younger generation—if you are a woman or care for women, this book is for you. The truth is that as much as women may differ, we are very much alike when it comes to how nutrition affects our health. The earlier you start paying attention to the lifelong *process* that is your nutritional health, the better. But remember two things: You're never too old to start, and even small changes can add up to big benefits.

Over the past 100 years, we have discovered a lot about the relationship between diet and health. And with every new finding has come the confirmation that there is still so much more to learn. Controversies have raged, quieted and raged again. Through it all, however, one thing hasn't changed and isn't likely to: The bottom line when it comes to a healthy diet is balance, variety and moderation. Now and in the future, you won't go wrong making these principles your touchstone. Here's how they work:

◆ **Balance:** I encourage you to balance your diet by eating from a range of different categories of food like fruits, vegetables, grains, dairy products and lean meats. The Food Guide Pyramid (chapter 4) gives you a basic plan to follow. It's important to balance your diet to ensure that you get the optimal amount of carbohydrate, protein and fat. As you'll see, all these nutrients are essential to your health.

In terms of physical activity, I urge you to balance your activity among three categories: aerobic exercise, strength training and stretching. Each one has distinct health benefits (see chapter 6).

♦ **Variety:** Within each broad food category, I recommend that you enjoy a variety of different foods—lots of different fruits, vegetables and grains; an assortment of dairy products; different kinds of lean meat and fish. Variety is important for two reasons: First, no single food contains all the essential mironutrients—the vitamins, minerals and other compounds your body needs to function smoothly and prevent disease. The greater the variety of foods you consume, the more vital nutrients you'll ingest. Second, variety is more fun and helps you keep your diet balanced. For example, if the only vegetable you ever eat is carrots, it's likely you'll get bored and end up skipping vegetables altogether. But if you stimulate your taste buds with a variety of vegetables, you're more likely to stick with a balanced diet.

The same holds true for exercise. For example, no one strength-training exercise or stretch does it all. But doing a variety of these exercises will help you be strong, toned and flexible all over. Variety also fights boredom in exercise—one of the main reasons people don't stick with a program.

♦ **Moderation:** By eating moderately, you maintain the flexibility you need to enjoy a variety of foods and to reap their healthy benefits. Eating moderately also helps you stay within an optimal calorie range for maintaining your healthy weight. In exercise, moderation is the key to avoiding injury. Following a reasonable exercise program that builds gradually over time also will help you stick with the program. Too much too fast leads to burnout.

Although you can read any chapter in *The American Dietetic Association Guide to Women's Nutrition for Healthy Living* as an independent piece, I urge you to start at the beginning and move through the total process with me. Here's a road map for the journey we'll take.

◆ CHAPTER 1: THEN AND NOW . . . AND YOU

In chapter 1, we'll take a brief historical look at women's health. I included this information because I think it's important to understand how far we have come and how difficult the road has been. When I first learned about the history of women's health and women in health care I was shocked, saddened and outraged. But most of all, I was proud of what we have accomplished, grateful to the pioneering women who fought and continue to fight for change, and hopeful for the future.

◆ CHAPTER 2: WOMEN AND DISEASE

The American Dietetic Association's Nutrition and Health Campaign for Women focuses on women's unique vulnerability to five diseases: breast cancer, heart disease, osteoporosis, diabetes and obesity. In chapter 2, we'll consider these diseases and talk about their risk factors and causes. We'll also explore the role of nutrition in prevention and treatment and talk about the direction of current research. When you see how many diseases share risk factors, I think you will understand why it's important to make *total* health your goal.

◆ CHAPTER 3: THE STAGES OF A WOMAN'S LIFE

After you finish this chapter, I hope you will have a new appreciation for nutritional health as a process that occurs across your life span. Although each stage of life comes with its own nutrition and health imperatives, there is a cumulative benefit to taking charge of your nutritional health sooner rather than later. This chapter also explains the interplay of estrogen and nutrition throughout your life cycle.

◆ CHAPTER 4: YOUR NUTRITION TOOL KIT

Some of you will be familiar with the three tools discussed in this chapter—the Dietary Guidelines, the Food Guide Pyramid and the food label. But chances are you've never seen them presented quite like this. Once you know how they work *together*, you'll have a nutrition tool kit that makes following a balanced diet—filled with variety and seasoned with moderation—as easy as one, two, three.

The second part of this chapter dispels some myths about, and is a primer on, what we know so far about antioxidants and phytochemicals.

◆ CHAPTER 5: LIFESTYLE "WEAR AND TEAR"

If you live a stress-free life, have never experienced negative feelings about your weight, have never had a food craving, and have never been on a diet—you can skip this chapter. If you are like most women, however, you will recognize yourself in these pages. But what you may not realize is how stress, negative body image and chronic dieting can wreak havoc on your nutritional health and your immunity to illness.

◆ CHAPTER 6: WHAT YOU CAN DO

In light of women's unique health needs, this chapter outlines four strategies you can put into action today, regardless of your age.

They're not a quick fix. They're not a diet plan. They are a path toward fundamental positive change in your nutritional health. These concise, realistic action steps not only target the prevention and treatment of breast cancer, heart disease, osteoporosis, diabetes and obesity, they also enhance your overall health and well-being. Adopt any one of the strategies and you'll be taking a significant step toward safeguarding your health. Incorporate all four into your life and you'll benefit from the power of their synergy.

CHAPTER 1

Then and Now . . . and You

Today, it's not unusual to see a report about women's health on the nightly news or to read a magazine article about how a particular disease affects both men and women. We're not surprised to hear about dollars being allocated to women's health research, nor are we hard-pressed to find a female doctor.

But it wasn't always so. Although women traditionally have been identified with nurturing and healing, we haven't always occupied level ground with men in medical treatment or practice. In fact, the story of women's health so far has been a dramatic one, with triumphs and setbacks all along the way.

THEN . . .

Writers such as Barbara Ehrenreich, Deirdre English and Jeanne Achterberg have chronicled the history of women's health. Looking back, we see that women often played a very important role in the health of society. In ancient myths from around the world, it was women who knew nature's secrets of life and death. And it was women who could practice the "magical" art of healing, which was considered a divine function. Ancient deities often were depicted as nurturing, healing mothers. As long as the reigning deity of a particular culture was feminine, women could practice the healing arts freely. But when the cultural focus shifted to a male god, women were given less access to education and their roles as healers diminished.

In ancient Greece—when reverence for the goddess Athena was at its pinnacle—women such as Helen of Troy and the Oracles of Delphi were renowned healers. Some scholars believe ancient Greek women were responsible for the surgical techniques and therapeutics that made Greek medicine the most advanced of its era. But by the time Aristotle and Hippocrates—the so-called fathers of medicine—the power of the goddesses had diminished and women were no longer respected as healers.

During the Dark Age in Europe, women healers worked mainly through informal networks. Eventually, they were forbidden to practice any kind of healing, not because they lacked knowledge, but because of the belief that women had powerful secret remedies and could intervene with the demonic supernatural. The penalty for practicing healing was death or imprisonment. During the 1500s, tens of thousands of women in France, Germany, Italy and England were hanged or burned at the stake as witches for violating the ban. It is difficult to believe, but it was only 221 years ago—in 1775—that the last witch was hanged in Germany.

During the Scientific Revolution, the practice of medicine changed dramatically. The body was regarded as a collection of parts that could be studied independently. Practitioners believed that nature could be dominated by science, reason and objectivity. In this vision of reality, women's link to nature and their supposed magical healing powers simply had no value.

Jumping ahead to America in the nineteenth century, we find a resurrection of women's traditional holistic perspective on health and health care. Disillusioned with the contemporary invasive approach to medicine, women turned once again to the ancient wisdom of nature as a healing resource. The Popular Health

Movement of the nineteenth century, which was led largely by women, advocated a healthy body and mind through nutrition, exercise, sunshine, fresh air, water and clean living.

By the late 1800s, women were being admitted to previously all-male medical schools and were graduating with honors. Soon, however, the largely male American Medical Association claimed that salaries and doctors' prestige were diminishing because the profession was becoming too crowded. As a result, medical schools stopped approving applications for women.

The door to medical school may have been barred, but women are not that easy to outsmart—or to outflank. They blazed a new trail into health care. After 1900, women flourished in nursing. Perhaps the most famous nursing practitioner of the time was Florence Nightingale, the "lady with the lamp" and a heroine of the Crimean War.

As the twentieth century began, the Popular Health Movement had lost some of its vigor. But before fading away, it had laid a grassroots foundation for the emergence of the Suffrage Movement and had empowered women to move from practicing "domestic health" to pursuing careers in professional health care.

Now . . .

By the late 1960s and early 1970s, women began to seek equality in education and the workplace. Today, women earn more than half of all bachelor's and master's degrees. Of the fifty-six million jobs created over the last thirty years, women have filled 64 percent. And the number of businesses owned by women is growing twice as fast as the number owned by men, increasing 43 percent from 1987 to 1992.

Like an echo from the past, health issues provided a catalyst for this progress. Early on, women's reproductive health served to coalesce the modern feminist movement. In 1969, Barbara Seaman's *The Doc-*

tors' Case Against the Pill raised the national consciousness and sparked congressional hearings on the safety of early birth control pills. Today, seventy-five years after women won the right to vote and twenty-five years after the birth of modern feminism, health has once again become a unifying issue for women. Today's focus on women's health and on equality in research, prevention and care has far-reaching ramifications for all people. With this renewed interest in women's health comes a return to traditional values that emphasize disease prevention, wellness and the health of the total person.

The Women's Health Initiative represents a giant step forward in this new era for women's health. A fourteen-year, $625-million research effort, the Initiative will study approximately 150,000 women and will shed light on the prevention and treatment of heart disease, cancer and osteoporosis. The women's Health Initiative is the largest clinical study ever undertaken by the National Institutes of Health (NIH). Women have traveled a long, hard and often circuitous route to arrive at this critical point. Prior to the Initiative, women were regularly excluded from clinical trials. But thanks to the leadership of committed, determined women of vision like former NIH director Bernadine Healy, M.D., who wrote the foreword for this book, we can now collect the data vital to understanding women's unique health needs.

THE SEARCH FOR RESEARCH

In the late 1980s, the Congressional Caucus for Women's Issues, a group of female U.S. congressional representatives, sounded an alarm: For years, it seems the medical research community had been ignoring women's unique health needs.

Women's health advocates discovered that research into diseases that affect both men and women often had included only male participants. Nevertheless, results from these one-sided studies were implicitly applied to women as well. So pervasive was this exclusion that only male rats were used for laboratory experiments!

Consider, for example, the Baltimore Longitudinal Study, one of the largest studies ever to examine the natural process of aging. It began in 1958 and for the first twenty years included no women, despite the fact that two-thirds of those over age sixty-five are women. (Currently, 50 percent of the participants in the study are women.)

Consider the Physicians' Health Study, better known as the "aspirin study." Conducted in 1988 by the Harvard Medical School and Boston's Brigham and Women's Hospital, this study concluded that taking an aspirin every other day may reduce the risk of heart disease. The study sample included 22,071 men but no women—even though heart disease is the number-one killer of women. Similarly, the 1982 Multiple Risk Factor Intervention Trial (aptly called "Mr. Fit"), a long-term study of lifestyle factors relating to cholesterol and heart disease, included 13,000 men and no women.

Researchers even went so far as to study the effect of estrogen as protection against heart disease—on men. And it doesn't stop there: They also explored the impact of obesity on the tendency for women to develop breast or endometrial cancer—using only male research subjects. As recently as 1987, only 13 percent of the NIH budget was spent to study diseases that exclusively, predominantly or more seriously affect women—for example, breast cancer, ovarian cancer and osteoporosis—or that have different risk factors or treatments in women—such as heart disease, depression and AIDS.

On the positive side is the ongoing Nurses' Health Study, an observational study of 120,000 female nurses that examines how lifestyle choices such as diet, exercise and smoking affect women's health. It was this study that finally confirmed estrogen's heart-protective benefits in women. And questions raised by the Nurses' Study clearly underscore the need for more aggressive women's health research.

Revelations about the women's health research gap provided the impetus for a 1990 General Accounting Office (GAO) investigation that showed the NIH had done little to implement policies supportive of women's health. The GAO report ignited a firestorm of controversy, propelling women's health into the forefront among hot political issues. Laws passed in 1993 mandated an Office of Research on Women's Health within NIH. These laws also specify that studies not only must include women (when appropriate) but also must be conducted so that gender differences can be analyzed.

If you are interested in learning more about the history of gender bias in medical research, here are several books you can read:

◆ *The American Woman 1994–95: Where We Stand, Women and Health* (W. W. Norton, 1994), edited by Cynthia Costello and Anne J. Stone.
◆ *Outrageous Practices: The Alarming Truth About How Medicine Treats Women* (Fawcett Columbine, 1994), by Leslie Laurence and Beth Weinhouse.
◆ *Unequal Treatment: What You Don't Know About How Women Are Mistreated by the Medical Community* (Simon & Schuster, 1994), by Eileen Nechas and Denise Foley.

CLAIMING OUR POWER

Today, we have the economic and educational clout to avoid the mistakes and injustices of the past. In fact, because of our roles as caregivers and gatekeepers, there is growing recognition that the health of women is critical to the well-being of men and children as well.

As family caregivers, we influence the health of our loved ones in a number of ways. For example, three-quarters of all family health-care decisions are made or significantly influenced by women. Women also initiate 90 percent of all calls to physician-referral and health-information services. For many women, the role of unpaid caregiver for an aging parent or in-law has been added to their traditional roles. Approximately seven million Americans are looking after an aging parent or relative. You may not be surprised to hear that three out of four of these caregivers are women.

In terms of dollars, women themselves are the greatest consumers of health care. We make significantly more physician visits than men and are hospitalized more often. We also account for three-fourths of today's long-term-care patients—not surprising when you consider that women's average life expectancy is almost eighty years, which is about seven years longer than men's.

But even though women are living longer in general—and longer than men, in particular—we are not necessarily living better. Women suffer from more illnesses, particularly chronic diseases, than men do. We also experience poorer health outcomes and greater disability than do men. The following statistics bring women's vulnerability into sharp focus.

- Heart disease is the number-one killer and disabler of America's women. Some 245,000 women die of heart disease each year.
- Cancer is the leading cause of premature death among women. 250,000 women die of cancer each year—46,000 of them from breast cancer.
- Osteoporosis affects more than twenty-five million Americans—twenty million, or 80 percent of them, are women.
- Six and a half million American women are afflicted with diabetes. Approximately 60 percent of the newly diagnosed cases of diabetes are in women, with a disproportionate incidence in minority women.
- One-third of U.S. women are overweight.

As you read this book, I hope you will also gain a deeper understanding of how what you eat affects the prevention and treatment of breast cancer, heart disease, osteoporosis, obesity and diabetes. Nutrition is probably the single biggest factor in the health and well-being of a woman at any stage of her life. For example, for some time we've known about the critical role of calcium in osteo-porosis prevention and treatment. Now, we are discovering more about the value of calcium intake over a lifetime and the important ways calcium interacts with other nutrients, with drug therapy, with estrogen and with exercise.

Similarly, it's no secret that high blood cholesterol is a risk factor for heart disease, but now we are learning more about how women's cholesterol-related risk differs from men's. We're also un-raveling the complexities of obesity—a disease in itself as well as a risk factor for heart disease, diabetes and certain cancers in women. And while we continue to look for the elusive link between dietary fat and breast cancer, we're discovering more about the cancer-fighting properties of antioxidants and other compounds found in fruits, vegetables and grains.

As researchers continue to explore the frontiers of women's health, you can take action now to protect yourself from some of the diseases that take a particularly high toll on women. You may not be able to change some of your risk factors—like age or hered-ity—but you can change how you eat. It is my sincere wish that in the pages that follow you find the inspiration, confidence and guid-ance you need to take charge of your nutritional health.

CHAPTER 2

Women and Disease

 $\mathcal{L}$iving a long life sounds good in theory, but it can be a mixed blessing. What really counts is living a long and *healthy* life. That's no easy task for women. Although they outlive men by about seven years, women are particularly vulnerable to an array of chronic diseases that can diminish their quality of life. In this chapter, we are going to look at five of the most common diseases that afflict women: breast cancer, heart disease, diabetes, obesity and osteoporosis. Each one has a strong link to nutrition.

We don't have all the answers about what causes these diseases, but we do know a number of the risk factors involved. Some risk factors are inherited and, consequently, can't be changed. Others, however, have to do with lifestyle and behavior choices that you can control. As medical practice becomes more prevention oriented, some experts predict that nutrition will be recognized as one of the most important controllable risk factors for disease.

Having certain risk factors doesn't necessarily mean that you are going to get a particular disease. It does mean you have a predisposition toward that disease and should strive to reduce your risk. For example, early menopause is a risk factor for osteoporosis, but early menopause itself does not *cause* osteoporosis. You can't stop menopause, but taking hormone replacement therapy, exercising more and making sure you get enough calcium can lower its impact as a risk factor.

A link to nutrition is not the only common thread running through the five diseases we're focusing on here. Breast cancer, heart disease, diabetes, obesity and osteoporosis are also influenced by estrogen. We've been hearing a lot about estrogen lately because of the benefits of hormone replacement therapy for some women. Estrogen, a multipurpose hormone, maintains the lining of the uterus and the vagina, stimulates growth of mammary tissue in the breast, preserves the elasticity of blood vessels, influences cholesterol production in the liver, inhibits bone loss and helps regulate body temperature.

Early in a woman's life, estrogen makes her more resistant to infection—more "immunologically talented." Researchers don't know exactly how the link between hormones and immunity works, but they do know that certain immune cells have estrogen receptors. But estrogen lets women down as they age. Eventually, women become more susceptible to autoimmune diseases like lupus in which the body attacks itself. Another irony of estrogen is that while it protects against some diseases—heart disease and osteoporosis, for example—it can be a detriment in others, like breast cancer. Researchers continue to explore the many facets of estrogen, including its relationship to nutrition.

BREAST CANCER

According to the American Cancer Society, breast cancer strikes an estimated 180,000 women yearly, resulting in 46,000 deaths—a third of all cancer deaths in women. Although it is not the deadliest of diseases that strike women (overall, heart disease has that dubious distinction), breast cancer is the most feared—in large part because it gets so much publicity. As one researcher put it, the breast as a symbol of femininity, sexuality and motherhood has much more emotional leverage than, say, the colon.

Breasts are a very visible part of a woman's personal identity. Consequently, many women experience real fear upon hearing that ominous statistic "One in eight women will develop breast cancer." But remember this: "One in eight" is a *lifetime* risk. The older you

---

What "One in Eight" Really Means

Breast Cancer Risk

By age 25:	one woman in 19,608 has developed breast cancer
By age 30:	one in 2,525
By age 35:	one in 622
By age 40:	one in 217
By age 45:	one in 93
By age 50:	one in 50
By age 55:	one in 33
By age 60:	one in 24
By age 65:	one in 17
By age 70:	one in 14
By age 75:	one in 11
By age 80:	one in 10
By age 85:	one in 9
Over age 85:	one in 8

It is important to remember two facts about these statistics: The "one in eight" risk for breast cancer is a *lifetime* risk, and developing breast cancer doesn't mean dying of the disease. The fatality risk is much lower: one in thirty by age ninety. You might be surprised to learn that your lifetime risk for developing other diseases is actually much greater: one in three for heart disease; one in two for osteoporosis; one in six for skin cancer.

---

are, the higher the likelihood that you have had breast cancer (one in 50 women by age 50, as noted in the sidebar), but the lower the likelihood that you will develop it. Between 12 percent and 20 percent of newly diagnosed breast cancers are in the very early stage and rarely lead to death.

All cancers, breast or otherwise, share one common trait: They are an invasive, uncontrolled growth of abnormal cells. It is not clear what causes cancer; recent research suggests that 65 percent of all cancer deaths are related to lifestyle—smoking, diet and lack of exercise. Although the disease may not manifest itself until later in life, its causes may date back to childhood.

Researchers have called the female breasts a "dynamic phenomenon," because of the many changes they undergo. Breast tissue changes with each menstrual cycle, pregnancy and lactation. Breasts even continue to change after menopause in ways medical science is just beginning to understand.

Who's at Risk?

A number of risk factors for breast cancer cluster around the hormone estrogen. They include early age at menarche (before twelve), late age at menopause (after fifty-five), no full-term pregnancies or late age at first birth (after thirty). All these risk factors involve repeated, long-term exposure of breast cells to estrogen. Because estrogen causes breast cells to multiply, the more your breasts are exposed to estrogen, the greater the chance for the kind of cellular accident that can lead to cancer.

If you are thinking about hormone therapy after menopause, consider that some studies have shown a slight risk of breast cancer associated with estrogen replacement. You may decide that the heart and bone health benefits of hormone replacement therapy (HRT) outweigh this risk. But if you have a strong family history of breast cancer, your physician may advise against HRT. In that case, you might be a candidate for a drug that mimics the positive attributes of estrogen without the negative effects. Major pharmaceutical companies are currently researching these estrogen analogs.

Having a mother or daughter with breast cancer is also a risk, but heredity accounts for only 5 percent to 10 percent of all cases—mostly among women under fifty. Two breast cancer genes, BRCA-1 and BRCA-2, have been discovered. One or both genes are thought to be implicated in as many as 25 percent of breast cancers diagnosed before age thirty. A third gene, known as ATM, increases a person's risk for a number of cancers, including breast cancer.

By age seventy, 85 percent of women who inherit one defective BRCA-1 gene will develop breast cancer. A similar proportion of women with a BRCA-2 mutation also develop breast cancer. If there is a suspicion of hereditary breast cancer in your family, you can have a blood test to screen for a defective BRCA-1 gene. But before testing you, your physician will want to test someone in your family with diagnosed breast cancer to confirm the genetic link. Before you undergo testing, it's a good idea to talk with a genetic counselor about your options should the test be positive.

What Can You Change?

Granted, you can't change your genetic makeup, nor can you do much about your reproductive cycles. But you can change the way you eat and exercise, and that can have a real impact on your breast health.

Much controversy exists about the role of dietary fat in breast cancer. You have probably heard conflicting reports in the media. Numerous studies comparing breast cancer rates in various countries show a clear link to a high-fat diet. An analysis of twelve different studies seems to confirm this link, But findings from the much publicized Nurses' Health Study show no relationship between fat and breast cancer.

It is difficult to know whom and what to believe. I am convinced—

as are a number of other nutrition professionals—that there is a link between dietary fat and breast cancer. We have yet to uncover it conclusively for several reasons. For example, we have not studied the effect of very low fat diets—15 percent to 20 percent of total calories. Or, since a high-fat diet is also high in calories, perhaps calories are actually the culprit. It also may be that the connection is not so much about current diet as it is about diet early in life when breasts are forming. This theory could explain why breast cancer rates are high in the U.S. despite the fact that fat consumption has dropped. Perhaps not enough time has passed to see the effect.

Obesity has been implicated in breast cancer, especially in postmenopausal women, and it's common knowledge that a high-fat diet contributes to obesity. A National Cancer Institute study suggests that if you're over fifty, relatively heavy and have gained more than ten pounds in the last decade, your risk of breast cancer might be three times as high as a thinner woman whose weight has remained stable. In fact, excess weight might be what tips the balance toward breast cancer in a woman who might have remained free of the disease for years to come.

Obesity's link to breast cancer may involve estrogen. Because fat cells produce estrogen, overweight women have higher levels of the hormone. Women with extra weight in the abdominal area (an apple-shaped versus a pear-shaped body) are at even greater risk because they tend to have higher insulin levels—another potential promoter of breast cancer.

Particularly exciting research is being done in Canada on the effect of a low-fat diet on the density of breast tissue. The National Cancer Institute has found that breast density increases the risk of cancer. We also know that high density of breast tissue makes it very difficult for mammography to detect abnormalities.

The Women's Health Initiative is looking at postmenopausal breast cancer and the effect of a low-fat diet that is high in fruits, vegetables and grains. There is some evidence that a diet rich in vegetables and fruit may lower the risk of breast cancer. The protective effect may not arise from any one nutrient, but rather from a combination of nutrients and other food components.

The obesity–breast cancer connection is not only an adult phenomenon. Childhood weight patterns can also have an effect on breast cancer. If you have a young daughter or granddaughter, remember that her present diet and exercise habits could have a lifelong effect on her breast health. We'll be seeing a lot of research on this connection in the years to come. One area involves the impact of weight on age of menarche (the onset of menstruation). A girl must have a certain percentage of body fat for menstruation to begin. Consequently, girls who are overweight experience earlier menarche than girls who weigh less. The sooner a girl begins menstruating, the greater her lifelong exposure to estrogen.

Another major topic of discussion in breast health is the effect of alcohol. This subject is controversial because there is some evidence that alcohol in moderation can be heart healthy. But one of the reasons alcohol is good for heart health may be the very same reason it's not beneficial for breast health: Alcohol apparently increases estrogen production. As few as two drinks a day may increase breast cancer risk by 40 percent. Research on this area is ongoing. For now, it's probably wise to limit alcohol consumption to one drink a day. If you don't drink, it's advisable not to start.

Like diet, exercise is something you can control. And at least one study has shown that women under age forty who exercise about four hours per week were 58 percent less likely to develop breast cancer than inactive women. You probably won't be surprised to hear that, once again, the connection appears to be estrogen. Habitual exercise makes women ovulate later in their cycle, reducing the amount of time the body is exposed to estrogen. Excessive exercise also suppresses ovulation. Without ovulation, less estrogen is produced.

Of all the strategies you can use to fight breast cancer, perhaps the most important is early detection. When caught early, breast cancer is highly treatable. About 95 percent of women with small, localized tumors will survive and live healthy, normal lives. Early

When to Have a Mammogram

According to the American Cancer Society, women age fifty and older should have a mammogram every year. Studies have shown that annual mammography reduces breast cancer deaths by an average of 30 percent in this age group.

Between ages forty and fifty, women should have a mammogram every year or two if they are at average risk for breast cancer. Although there is some controversy over the effectiveness of annual mammography for women between ages forty and fifty, a number of studies do support the effectiveness of yearly testing. If you are in this age group, consult with your physician about your particular risk factors and needs.

Young women have dense breast tissue that makes it difficult to detect tumors, so for women under age forty, mammography is likely to be less informative.

Improved breast cancer detection methods include high-definition ultrasound, which may be able to reduce surgical biopsies by 40 percent. Eventually, a new blood test used in conjunction with mammograms and clinical breast exams may detect tumor recurrence in some breast cancer patients. And on a really high-tech note, in the "missiles to mammograms" program, major medical centers are testing imaging technologies used by the Central Intelligence Agency and the Department of Defense. If we can detect water on the moon, we should be able to better detect breast cancer.

If you find a suspicious breast lump or if a routine mammogram and/or ultrasound suggest an abnormality, your doctor will probably recommend a biopsy. Biopsies range from needle procedures done under local anesthesia to removal of the lump under general anesthesia. The more tissue removed, the lower the chance that cancer cells will escape unnoticed. Fortunately, however, advances in testing mean less and less tissue is needed to identify cancer cells and their exact makeup.

detection depends on regular self-examinations plus yearly clinical breast exams and mammography as appropriate for your age (see sidebar). If you are at risk with a strong family history of breast cancer, your doctor may suggest more frequent monitoring.

Points to Remember

To improve your breast health:

◆ **Follow a low-fat diet.**
◆ **Increase your exercise.**
◆ **Maintain a healthy weight.**
◆ **Have regular mammograms and clinical breast exams.**

HEART DISEASE

Before we take a closer look at heart disease, let's clear up some confusion over definitions. Both heart disease and stroke are known as *cardiovascular diseases,* which are disorders of the heart and blood vessel system. *Coronary heart disease* or *coronary artery disease* is a disease of the heart's blood vessels, which leads to heart attack—meaning a blocked artery prevents oxygen and nutrients from reaching the heart muscle. Heart attacks are sometimes called *myocardial infarctions.* In a *stroke,* or brain attack, a blocked artery prevents enough blood from getting to part of the brain or, in some cases, a brain hemorrhage occurs. High blood pressure (hypertension), angina (chest pain) and rheumatic heart disease are also cardiovascular diseases.

All heart and blood vessel diseases combined claim more than 479,000 women's lives each year. All forms of cancer take just about half that number of female lives. Although women are susceptible to the full range of cardiovascular diseases, they are particularly vulnerable to heart disease. About 245,000 U.S. women die from heart disease each year. By comparison, about 46,000 women die of breast cancer annually.

Despite the overwhelming statistics, many women still think breast cancer is their gender's leading cause of death. Heart disease is still thought to be primarily a man's disease—the "widow maker," as it has been called. Many women know how to prevent and care for heart disease in their fathers, husbands and sons but don't have a clue how to protect themselves.

Heart Attack: A Woman's Warning Signs

Men often exhibit "textbook" symptoms of heart attack, while women do not. Why? Because the textbooks were written about men! Consequently, it comes as no surprise that almost nine out of ten doctors surveyed by Gallup in 1995 said that heart disease symptoms are the same in men and women. The classic (that is, male) signs of a heart attack are severe chest pain, shortness of breath, numbness, pain or tingling in the left arm or jaw, disorientation and sweating.

The truth is that we are still learning the classic symptoms for women. We do know that chest pain is less likely to signal heart disease in women than in men. Women sometimes have intermittent pain or symptoms. They often experience shortness of breath, nausea, unexplained heartburn or profound fatigue. Women are more likely to ignore or downplay these warning signs because they simply don't expect to have heart disease. Studies show that women typically wait four to eight hours before seeking help. Men, however, usually seek help in about an hour.

Once you reach middle age, you should pay especially close attention to potential heart attack symptoms. Men are more likely than women to experience acute and dramatic heart attacks, but women are more likely to have chronic heart disease that worsens over time. This may be one reason why heart

---

surgery is riskier for women. By the time the need is recognized, women are too sick to benefit. Take all chest pain, even pain that comes and goes, very seriously.

Even if you have no family history of heart disease and no known risk factors, it is a good idea to have baseline resting electrocardiogram and evaluation before age forty-five. Traditional treadmill stress tests are less accurate in women than in men. Stress *echo*cardiograms, which use ultrasound rather than electric monitoring, are more accurate in both men and women. Angiography, the gold standard for diagnosing heart disease, is also accurate in both men and women. Unfortunately, only half as many women as men are referred for this test.

Although heart disease generally strikes women after age sixty-five—about a decade later than in men—that doesn't mean younger women are not at risk. More than 20,000 women under age sixty-five die of heart attacks each year, and almost a third of them are under age fifty-five. One very frightening reality is that in more than two-thirds of women who die suddenly of heart disease, there were no previous symptoms. And of those women who survive a heart attack, more than 40 percent will die within a year—compared to fewer than 30 percent of male victims. For older women the picture is especially grim; they are twice as likely as men to die from a heart attack within just a few weeks of the attack.

Possibly related to this bleak outlook is the fact that fewer women than men are referred by their physicians for cardiac rehabilitation, which includes nutrition and exercise counseling. In fact, after hospitalization, only 20 percent of all patients entering structured rehabilitation programs are women. After a heart attack women also suffer more depression, anxiety and guilt feelings about their illness than do men.

It is ironic, though, that despite this gloomy outlook, women actually do very well in cardiac rehab—if and when they get there. Some research indicates that women may be able to reverse heart disease without making the substantial changes in diet and exercise typically required of men. Women also do a better job of following the advice of health professionals and sticking with their programs over time.

Who's at Risk?

Researchers have identified an array of risk factors for heart disease. Men and women share some; others are unique to women. Some can't be changed; others can.

Age and heredity (family history and race) are risk factors none of us—men or women—can change. Heart disease often runs in families. For women, the chances of developing heart disease increase with age due in large part to estrogen. We'll examine that connection in more detail later. African-American women are at greater risk than Caucasian women because they tend to have higher blood pressure levels and a greater number are overweight.

An Aspirin a Day?

You may have heard that taking aspirin every day can help prevent heart attacks. In 1988, the Harvard Physicians' Health Study did show that taking a small amount of aspirin (one-half to one tablet) each day could lower heart attack risk—in men. Because women were excluded from this research, no one was really sure if they also could benefit from a daily dose of aspirin.

Later, researchers analyzed data collected from women in the Nurses' Health Study. Results suggest that aspirin protects women from heart disease, too. But because aspirin can cause gastrointestinal bleeding and is known to increase the risk of stroke (from hemorrhage), you and your doctor should carefully assess your total health profile before adding aspirin to your daily preventive health regimen. Meanwhile, research continues on the effect of aspirin on women's heart disease risk.

What Can You Change?

Smoking is the greatest single preventable cause of heart disease and death. Women who smoke have twice the risk of heart attack compared to nonsmoking women. It is very disturbing to see smoking on the rise among teenage girls, who often use it as a weight control measure. If you don't smoke, don't start. If you smoke, quit. Keep trying. Don't give up. If your loved ones smoke, urge them to quit.

High blood pressure increases your risk of heart disease as well as stroke and kidney disease. Nearly half of all women over age fifty-five have high blood pressure. Hypertension occurs nearly three times more often among overweight adults than among adults at a healthy weight. It's often called the "silent killer" because most people who have it don't feel sick. If your blood pressure consistently measures 140/90 or higher, you are at risk. Talk to your doctor about controlling your blood pressure with weight loss and/or medication.

Diabetes is another major heart attack risk factor that is linked to obesity. More than 80 percent of people with diabetes die of some form of cardiovascular disease. Your risk of diabetes increases about twofold if you are mildly overweight, fivefold if you're moderately overweight, and tenfold if you are obese. The most common form of diabetes, type 2 (often called adult-onset diabetes), affects many more women than men after age forty-five, and having diabetes increases a woman's risk of heart disease more than it does a man's. Although premenopausal women are protected against heart disease by estrogen, diabetes eliminates estrogen's protective effect.

Even without high blood pressure or diabetes, obesity by itself increases the likelihood of having a heart attack. Again, body shape is important. The risk of heart attack is even greater when fat is mostly in the abdomen (apple-shaped body) rather than the hips and thighs (pear-shaped body). This central-body fat is believed to adversely affect blood cholesterol. Even modest weight gains in adulthood can raise a woman's chance of heart attack. Findings from the Nurses' Health Study suggest that weighing even ten to fifteen pounds more than your ideal weight can be risky.

High blood cholesterol is another major risk factor for heart disease, but most of the research in this area has been done on men. Findings from these studies can't be applied directly to women because estrogen has such a big influence on women's cholesterol numbers. What complicates the picture even more is the fact that levels of total cholesterol, LDL ("bad" cholesterol), HDL ("good" cholesterol) and triglycerides probably mean different things in men and women. Consequently, the results must be interpreted differently for each gender.

For example, high total cholesterol and LDL levels may be less dangerous to women than to men. A low HDL level (below 60), however, is a more serious threat in women and a strong predictor of heart disease. A high triglyceride level (above 400) is also more predictive of heart-disease risk in women than in men—especially if HDL is low, too. Some cardiologists don't worry about a man's triglyceride level until it reaches 400. For women, though, a level as high as 190 is a risk. High triglycerides are also related to the risk for diabetes. (For more about cholesterol, see chapter 4.)

When you have your cholesterol tested (start around age twenty), be sure to ask your doctor for *all* your blood-fat values, including triglycerides. It's called a *fractionated* cholesterol test. Your results should be monitored closely.

Recommended Cholesterol and Triglyceride Guidelines for Women

	Desirable	Borderline/ High Risk	High Risk
Total cholesterol	below 200	200–239	240 and above
LDL cholesterol	below 130	130–159	160 and above
HDL cholesterol	60 and above	59–34	35 and below
Triglycerides	below 190	190–399	400 and above

Estrogen levels affect your blood fats throughout life (see chapter 3). As estrogen levels drop at menopause, women's risk for heart disease grows dramatically. The evidence is clear that hormone replacement therapy reduces this risk. One reason is that both estrogen and estrogen-progestin combinations lower LDL cholesterol levels and increase HDL levels by 10 percent to 15 percent. This benefit plus estrogen's positive effect on bone health make hormone replacement therapy an attractive choice for many women. But taking estrogen does slightly increase the risk of breast cancer. The decision to take estrogen or not is a difficult call, and you'll want to make an informed decision. Discuss your family history along with the pros and cons of treatment with your physician.

Before menopause, your HDL level will be controlled in large part by heredity. Some women, however, can boost their HDL level by losing weight, especially in the abdominal area, and by doing regular aerobic exercise. Dozens of studies have shown that exercise is great all-around heart disease prevention. In fact, sedentary people who begin a regular exercise program can reduce their risk by 35 percent to 55 percent.

We're also learning more and more every day about micronutrients like antioxidants. In the case of heart disease, for example, re-

searchers believe that antioxidants, especially vitamin E, keep cholesterol in the blood from oxidizing, which is like rusting or cor-
roding. Once oxidized, cholesterol is more likely to form fatty
deposits in the arteries that block blood flow. Consequently, lowering cholesterol by eating less saturated fat and dietary cholesterol
may well be only half the battle. Generous amounts of fruits and
vegetables provide the antioxidants needed to complete the picture. More than ever before, it is becoming clear why balance, variety and moderation are the watchwords of a healthy diet. We'll
explore more of this frontier in chapter 4.

Finally, we now know that getting enough of the B vitamin folic
acid in the diet is important for heart health. You may have heard
about the importance of folic acid in preventing neural tube birth
defects. Researchers have also found that folic acid lowers high levels of an amino acid called homocysteine. Findings from the Fram-
ingham Heart Study confirm that people with high homocysteine
levels are twice as likely as those with low levels to have clogged arteries. You need about 400 micrograms of folic acid daily. It's
found in a number of foods like orange juice, leafy greens and
beans. Beginning in 1998, folic acid will be added to enriched
bread and other grain products. We'll revisit this vitamin in chapter 4.

Points to Remember

To improve your heart health:

- ◆ **Don't smoke.**
- ◆ **Follow a low-fat diet.**
- ◆ **Eat more fruits and vegetables.**
- ◆ **Maintain a healthy weight.**
- ◆ **Monitor your blood cholesterol levels, especially HDL
  cholesterol and triglyceride levels.**
- ◆ **Consider hormone replacement therapy if appropriate.**

DIABETES

Diabetes kills approximately 90,000 women each year, about twice the number that succumb to breast cancer. Diabetes has gone by a number of different names, so let's sort out the nomenclature. *Insulin dependent diabetes mellitus,* as it was called, is usually diagnosed in young people. In the past, it was also called *juvenile diabetes.* Today, it's called *type 1* diabetes. In people with type 1 diabetes, the body virtually stops producing insulin, a hormone that regulates glucose (blood sugar), the main sugar that results from digesting food. Peo-

---

Diabetes Symptoms

These symptoms are commonly associated with type 1 diabetes. People with type 2 diabetes may have abnormal blood sugar for years without developing any symptoms.

- ◆ Frequent urination
- ◆ Unusual thirst
- ◆ Extreme hunger
- ◆ Unusual weight loss
- ◆ Extreme fatigue
- ◆ Irritability
- ◆ Frequent or recurring infections
- ◆ Blurred vision
- ◆ Cuts and bruises that are slow to heal
- ◆ Tingling or numbness in the hands and feet

If you experience any of these symptoms, consult your doctor. He or she may order diagnostic tests that measure the amount of sugar in your blood after an all-night fast. If this level is too high, you may be advised to take a glucose tolerance test, which measures blood glucose levels over a period of several hours.

All pregnant women are usually tested for gestational diabetes.

---

ple with type 1 diabetes have to monitor their diet and exercise. Drugs to treat type 1 diabetes are in development but for now, people with this disease must inject insulin daily. Type 1 diabetes accounts for only 5 percent to 10 percent of diabetes and is not on the rise.

Type 2 diabetes, however, is increasing, and it is the kind of diabetes we are going to concentrate on. Type 2 diabetes was also called *noninsulin dependent diabetes mellitus*. Anyone can get type 2 diabetes, but it typically affects older people, which is why it used to be labeled *adult-onset diabetes*. If you have type 2 diabetes, your body still produces insulin, often a lot of it, but your cells are resistant to it. Consequently, glucose doesn't enter your cells as it should (where it is used for energy). Instead, it remains circulating in your blood. As type 2 diabetes worsens, the pancreas becomes unable to secrete an adequate amount of insulin.

Left untreated, diabetes can lead to kidney disease and failure, eye disease and blindness, circulatory problems (which can result in amputation of the legs or feet), heart disease and stroke. Premenopausal women's lower risk of heart disease is nullified by diabetes. Women with diabetes have a greater risk for both heart disease and stroke than do diabetic men. And diabetic women have a poorer prognosis after a heart attack than do men with diabetes.

Who's at Risk?

According to the American Diabetes Association, 60 percent of the new cases of diabetes are diagnosed in women. Approximately 6.5 million women in the United States have diabetes, but half of them don't know it and won't become aware until serious complications arise. African-American, Latina and Native American women are particularly vulnerable.

Nondiabetic pregnant women are at risk for *gestational* diabetes, which can lead to hypertension and toxemia (a dangerous complication characterized by generalized swelling, excess protein in the urine and hypertension). Women with gestational diabetes also are two to three times more likely to have higher birth weight babies and, as a result, more cesarean deliveries. Although blood sugar levels will return to normal after delivery, about half of women with gestational diabetes will develop type 2 diabetes later in life.

If you are over forty-five, overweight and get little exercise, you are a likely candidate for type 2 diabetes. Having a parent or sibling with diabetes also increases your risk. Before developing full-blown diabetes, you may have *impaired glucose tolerance* (IGT). About twenty million people have IGT, and most don't know it. Like diabetes, IGT is characterized by high blood glucose levels after meals—high enough, some scientists believe, to cause heart disease.

People with IGT are insulin resistant as well. Researchers believe that insulin resistance, which can be genetic as well as triggered by obesity, is a leading cause of diabetes and heart disease. As much as 10 percent to 25 percent of the population may be insulin resistant. Although insulin resistance has garnered a lot of media attention, may people don't understand what it really means.

Our body's cells are insulin resistant when they resist the message insulin is trying to give them—that is, to take in glucose from the blood to use as energy. When glucose can't enter our cells, it builds up in the bloodstream. The pancreas then excretes even more insulin to help the cells hear the message. That creates a double whammy: Too much glucose circulating in the blood not only causes tissue damage to the eyes, kidneys, nerves and heart but also leads to too much circulating insulin, which elevates triglycerides and blood pressure and lowers HDL "good" cholesterol, causing an increased risk for heart disease.

As an overweight person with insulin resistance gains even more weight, she eventually becomes unable to produce enough insulin. Her blood sugar will rise and she will become diabetic. Women with diabetes often have a blood fat profile that is similar to women with high risk for heart disease—that is, low HDL cholesterol and high triglycerides.

Some of the most exciting genetic research in diabetes and obesity is focusing on the communication breakdown that prevents cells from responding properly to insulin. There was a time in early human history when insulin resistance was a good thing. When the body needed fat stores to get through periods of famine, insulin resistance ensured that not all glucose was used for immediate energy. Some was stored as fat. But with today's ample food supply and sedentary lifestyle, insulin resistance is no longer beneficial.

What Can You Change?

Although there are no guarantees when it comes to preventing diabetes, there are some steps you can take to lower your risk. Maintaining a healthy weight is your single most important preventive strategy. Although not all obese people will develop diabetes, about 90 percent of people with diabetes are overweight. Again, apple-shaped people, those with weight around their middle, are more vulnerable than pear-shaped people, who store fat in their hips and thighs.

A New Look at Sugar

In 1994, the American Diabetes Association came out with new guidelines on the dietary management of diabetes. These revised guidelines suggest that 10 percent to 20 percent of calories should come from protein, less than 10 percent from saturated fat, up to 10 percent from polyunsaturated fat, and the remaining 60 percent to 70 percent from carbohydrates and monounsaturated fat.

The guidelines are just that: guidelines, not rules. If you have diabetes, you need to work with your physician and nutrition professional to design a dynamic, flexible plan that takes into account your unique needs, including other health risks.

Some people with diabetes, especially those who have low HDL cholesterol and high triglycerides, may benefit from a

---

diet that is lower in carbohydrates and higher in monounsaturated fat, like the fat in olive oil. The challenge, however, is not to increase *total* calorie intake when increasing monounsaturated fat. Otherwise, you'll gain weight.

Carbohydrates have also been reappraised. People with diabetes used to be told to avoid simple sugars—like those in sweets and soft drinks—in favor of complex carbohydrates found in starches like potatoes and rice. It was thought that simple sugars were more rapidly digested and therefore aggravated high blood sugar. Now it appears that a carbohydrate is a carbohydrate, no matter where it comes from. What is important is the total amount of carbohydrates consumed, not the type. Nevertheless, it's probably a good idea for people with diabetes to avoid eating a lot of sweets. The carbohydrates may be okay, but sweets tend to be high in fat and calories and low in other important nutrients like vitamins and minerals. In other words, they are not "nutrient dense." This is good advice for all women, not just those with diabetes.

The new guidelines also include a brief discussion of chromium. Since most people with diabetes are not chromium deficient, the guidelines maintain, chromium supplementation has no real benefit. But that's not what you've been hearing in the news, where it seems that chromium is a virtual cure for diabetes.

Studies have shown that chromium helps insulin transfer glucose into cells, which could benefit people who are insulin resistant and those who already have diabetes. But there's still a lot we don't know—like how much chromium is needed and how long the effect lasts. Currently, there is no solid evidence to recommend chromium supplements. But this is an important area of research and one that bears watching. For now, the best advice is to eat a variety of foods that include chromium, such as lean meat, eggs and whole grains.

If diabetes runs in your family and you're overweight, you are extremely vulnerable. According to findings from the Nurses' Health Study, a weight gain of more than eighteen to twenty-four pounds after age eighteen triples the risk of developing diabetes. When an overweight person loses weight, however, insulin resistance decreases, which usually lowers blood glucose levels. In chapter 6, we'll talk more about how to maintain a healthy weight.

Regular physical activity also helps prevent diabetes—regardless of your age or family history. Vigorous exercise promotes weight control and helps prevent insulin resistance. But even if you don't lose weight, exercise lowers blood sugar because it makes the muscles more sensitive to insulin and better able to absorb glucose. Exercise can also help people who already have type 2 diabetes to cut down or even eliminate the need for medication. Regular physical activity is also a known benefit in the prevention and treatment of heart disease, which is how most people with diabetes will die.

A low-fat diet rich in fruits and vegetables—the regimen that is known to lower the risk of some cancers and heart disease—may be helpful in preventing diabetes as well. We are not sure of the *direct* effect of this kind of diet on diabetes prevention, but we do know that a healthy diet is the key to reaching and maintaining a healthy weight. With obesity such a strong predictor of diabetes, it's easy to see why diet is an important prevention strategy.

If you already have diabetes and want to modify your diet to lose weight, be sure to consult with your physician and a nutrition professional. The American Diabetes Association recommends following a calorie-restricted diet, but within that plan there is a variety of fat and carbohydrate combinations (see sidebar A New Look at Sugar, page 34). It is important to remember that there is no such thing as a one-size-fits-all diet. You'll need some professional help developing a plan that suits your unique health needs and your lifestyle.

Points to Remember

To help avoid diabetes:

- ◆ **Maintain a healthy weight.**
- ◆ **Follow a low-fat diet.**
- ◆ **Increase your exercise.**

OBESITY

Obesity has become the nation's leading nutrition problem and is now recognized as a life-threatening disease. It is also a risk factor for a number of other diseases, including breast cancer, heart disease and diabetes.

Who's at Risk?

Obesity is on the rise, especially among women—particularly African-Americans and Latinas. According to U.S. government studies, a third of adults twenty to seventy-four years of age are overweight (or 20 percent above their desirable weight). Broken down by gender, that's 35 percent of women (thirty-two million) and 32 percent of men (twenty-six million). If we use the stricter World Health Organization indices to measure unhealthy weight, those percentages jump to 49 percent of women and 59 percent of men!

To a great extent, your genes determine whether you *can* become obese, but other influences—namely food and exercise—determine whether you *will* become obese and to what extent.

You've probably heard a lot about the various obesity genes scientists have discovered in mice over the past several years. The first one, designated *ob*, produces a hormonelike substance called leptin that helps the brain regulate appetite. The next discovery, *db*, is a gene that allows leptin to reduce appetite and crank up metabo-

Obesity vs. Overweight: What's the Difference?

Although these terms are used interchangeably, they do have distinct meanings. *Overweight* refers to an excess amount of *total* body weight—fat, bone, muscle and water. *Obesity* refers specifically to excess body fat. It is possible to be overweight without being obese. Think of an athlete who has a lot of muscle mass. It's also possible, but uncommon, to be obese without being overweight. A person may appear to be a normal weight, but that weight might be composed of a lot of fat and no muscle. In general, overweight people tend to be obese as well.

Body mass index (BMI) and weight-for-height tables are used to assess obesity. BMI is calculated by dividing weight in kilograms by height in meters and then squaring the result. The U.S. government's ongoing obesity task force uses a BMI of 27.8 for men and 27.3 for women to measure adult obesity. The World Health Organization uses a range of 25 to 29. A BMI between 19 and 25 is considered healthy.

Calculating Body Mass Index (BMI)

To determine your BMI, find your height (in inches) in the far-left column. Move across the row to your weight. The number on top of that column is your BMI.

Body Mass Index

Height (in.)	19	20	21	22	23	24	25	26	27	28	29	30	35	40
							Body Weight (lbs.)							
58	91	96	100	105	110	115	119	124	129	134	138	143	167	191
59	94	99	104	109	114	119	124	128	133	138	143	148	173	198
60	97	102	107	112	118	123	128	133	138	143	148	153	179	204
61	100	106	111	116	122	127	132	137	143	148	153	158	185	211
62	104	109	115	120	126	131	136	142	147	153	158	164	191	218
63	107	113	118	124	130	135	141	146	152	158	163	169	197	225
64	110	116	122	128	134	140	145	151	157	163	169	174	204	232
65	114	120	126	132	138	144	150	156	162	168	174	180	210	240
66	118	124	130	136	142	148	155	161	167	173	179	186	216	247
67	121	127	134	140	146	153	159	166	172	178	185	191	223	255
68	125	131	138	144	151	158	164	171	177	184	190	197	230	262
69	128	135	142	149	155	162	169	176	182	189	196	203	236	270
70	132	139	146	153	160	167	174	181	188	195	202	207	243	278
71	136	143	150	157	165	172	179	186	193	200	208	215	250	286
72	140	147	154	162	169	177	184	191	199	206	213	221	258	294
73	144	151	159	166	174	182	189	197	204	212	219	227	265	302
74	148	155	163	171	179	186	194	202	210	218	225	233	272	311
75	152	160	168	176	184	192	200	208	216	224	232	240	279	319
76	156	164	172	180	189	197	205	213	221	230	238	246	287	328

lism. Two additional genes produce proteins that regulate how fat is burned.

Although researchers have also located versions (called homologues) of all four of these genes within human DNA, they have not yet found the mutations that lead to obesity in people. Scientists believe that there are probably a number of interacting genes that affect appetite and weight in humans. Ongoing research is needed to sort out this genetic puzzle and to determine how diet and exercise interact with our genetic makeup.

Some experts maintain that we have a genetically determined "set point"—that is, a predetermined weight at which our bodies are happiest. The set point is likely to be an evolutionary tool humans developed to ensure that their fat levels remained constant during times of famine and plenty. Unfortunately, what was a protective mechanism thousands of years ago has become an obstacle to weight loss for some people today. The brain adjusts metabolism and influences behavior to maintain the body's set point. The set point mechanism is probably connected somehow to the *ob* and *db* genes and their messenger protein leptin.

Diet and exercise can move you away from your set point for a time, but they won't change the set point. In fact, it appears that set points aren't changeable in adulthood, but there may be a genetically programmed window of opportunity in childhood where the set point can be influenced by diet and exercise. If this theory proves true, it's one more reason to pay close attention to your daughters' and granddaughters' early eating and exercise habits.

You may have heard the term *brown fat*. Some animals, including humans, are born with special fat cells that burn glucose and release the energy as heat rather than storing the glucose as fat. These brown-fat cells help keep newborns warm. You may notice that an infant's back is warmer than the rest of her body. That warmth is coming from brown-fat cells acting like little heat engines. But these cells are turned off early in infancy—except in animals that hibernate because they need to produce heat to compensate for inactivity.

In humans, white-fat cells kick on to ensure a source of energy from stored fat. Obesity researchers are trying to find a way to reactivate our brown-fat cells. In mice missing a gene that helps regulate metabolism, energy is burned faster than it can be stored. Scientists believe this is the result of brown fat at work, but the challenge is translating these findings to humans.

All adults tend to gain weight from their mid thirties to their mid forties—women more so than men. Whereas men tend to level off, women keep on gaining well into their fifties. In fact, from age twenty-five to fifty-four women typically gain almost twice as much weight as men.

The situation is even more troubling among female children. There are three critical growth periods in a girl's life that can affect obesity in later years: gestation and early infancy, followed by ages five to seven and finally during adolescence. One in five teenagers and almost a third of six-to-eleven-year-olds are seriously overweight. During adolescence girls have a greater risk than boys of becoming obese and staying that way. A third of all fat women were obese in early adolescence, compared to only a tenth of obese adult men.

As far as its physical impact is concerned, obesity is a common but controllable risk factor for illness and death. It directly contributes to heart disease and complicates other diseases and other risk factors—such as insulin resistance, diabetes, hypertension, stroke, high cholesterol, and cancer. The more overweight you are and the longer you stay that way, the worse the effect.

What Can You Change?

What exactly causes obesity? On paper it looks simple: If the number of calories you eat exceeds the amount of energy you burn, you gain weight. What causes this imbalance between what you eat and what you burn is unclear. Yes, obesity tends to run in families, but we tend to share not only genes but eating and exercise habits as well. These lifestyle factors play an important role in determining

Apples and Pears

It's interesting that we use the names of foods to describe two particular styles of body fat distribution—apples and pears. If you tend to carry your weight in your waist and abdominal area, you're an apple. If your body fat is concentrated in the hip and thigh area, you're a pear. Women tend to be pears; men are more often apples.

Estrogen and testosterone influence this fat distribution. Premenopausal women accumulate fat in the lower body. But when estrogen levels fall at menopause and women gain weight, they tend to take on an apple shape. Premenopausal women who have more central body fat, more like men, have higher levels of the predominantly male hormone testosterone.

Although lower body fat isn't harmless, central body fat is more dangerous because it is more metabolically active. Consequently, apples tend to have lower HDL cholesterol and higher triglyceride levels as well as higher levels of insulin circulating in the blood, which can induce insulin resistance and promote diabetes. In addition, blood pressure is higher and the incidence of hypertension is greater in apple-shaped people. Some studies have shown that central body fat is more predictive of heart disease risk than overall body weight.

If your waist-hip ratio (WHR) is greater than 0.8, talk to your physician and nutrition professional about how to lower your risk. You can determine your WHR by dividing your waist measurement (at the area of smallest girth above your navel) by your hip measurement (at the largest horizontal girth between your waist and thighs). For example, if your waist measures 26 inches and your hips 36 inches, your WHR is 0.78 (26 ÷ 36 = 0.78).

weight. We can't change our genetic makeup, but we can change how we eat and exercise.

For example, we can alter the way we think about calories. Even though we are eating less dietary fat these days, we are consuming *more* calories—100 to 300 more calories per day over the past decade. That's enough to gain as much as thirty pounds a year! Loading up on low-fat and no-fat foods is not the way to maintain a healthy weight. The bottom line is: Calories still count.

We can change our exercise habits, too. As many as 40 percent of American adults are completely sedentary. Only about a third of adult women exercise frequently. And physical education is no longer a priority in many of our schools. According to government reports, fewer children, especially teens, are exercising regularly or strenuously.

Psychological factors can affect your weight by influencing your eating habits. You may eat not because you are hungry, but rather because you're stressed out, bored, depressed, sad, angry, or even happy. A significant number of obese people have a problem with binge eating. They eat large amounts of food at one time and feel they have no control. If this describes you, see a health professional immediately. You may have binge eating disorder and will need some special help to manage your weight.

The consequences of obesity affect not only your physical health, but your psychological health and social well-being, too. American society places a high value on physical appearance, especially on being thin. Obese people are often discriminated against in school, at work, in the job market and in social situations. For women, the negative body image associated with obesity, especially in female children and teens, can lead to eating disorders, self-esteem problems, depression and sexual dysfunction.

Maintaining a "healthy weight" is a relatively new idea based on a theory of diversity. Obesity has a number of causes and develops differently depending on age, gender, ethnicity and socioeconomics. Just as obesity is expressed differently in different people—for example, in body shape and related risk factors, so is healthy weight. Although you may match your neighbor in height and age, your healthy weight may not be the same as hers. The good news is that studies show even a loss of just 5% to 10% of body weight can lower blood pressure, blood sugar, cholesterol and triglycerides; boost HDL cholesterol; and increase self-esteem. Modest and gradual weight loss (about 1/2 to 1 pound per week) rather than a crash diet, can also help you succeed in keeping pounds off.

Before we leave this discussion of obesity, let me say that if you are jumping on the scale every morning and letting that number you see color your whole day in a negative way, stop. Stop "dieting" as well. Most people see a diet as a temporary way of life. They do it long enough to achieve results, then go back to their old eating habits—and gain back all the weight. Chapter 5 includes some more information on why diets don't work—plus a look at weight-loss drugs. In chapter 6, we'll talk about exercise and healthy weight management. As you continue to read this book, try to make a fundamental shift in the way you think about diet, exercise and weight. Make the healthy enjoyment of food your lifelong goal.

Points to Remember

How to maintain a healthy weight:

- ◆ **Remember that calories do count.**
- ◆ **Increase your exercise**
- ◆ **Stop dieting. Adopt a healthy eating attitude and a well-balanced diet.**

OSTEOPOROSIS

"I'm melting! I'm melting!" says the wicked witch in the *Wizard of Oz* as she slowly caves in upon herself. A woman with advanced osteoporosis may feel much the same way as her bones slowly weaken, as she shrinks in size and as she becomes painfully disfigured with "dowager's hump."

Osteoporosis has been called the "silent disease" not only because it can progress for years without any symptoms, but also because society has largely ignored it. We called it "brittle bone disease" and, until recently, largely accepted the crippling hip fractures it causes as an unfortunate part of aging.

Eight million people have osteoporosis, and another seventeen million are at risk. Of these twenty-five million victims, twenty million are women. By the year 2020, the number of Americans over age fifty will increase by 69 percent. Thus, millions of women will be entering a time in their lives when their risk of osteoporosis is high. For an elderly woman, the risk of hip fracture is as high as her combined chance of getting breast, uterine or ovarian cancer. And the inactivity that comes with that hip fracture can lead to serious complications, even death.

Before we examine the risk factors associated with osteoporosis, let's get a better idea about what this disease really means to women.

People with osteoporosis have a loss in bone tissue and bone strength. Bones are made of two types of tissue: an outer shell of dense bone called *cortical* and an inner honeycomb of spongy bone called *trabecular*. When you have osteoporosis, your cortical shell is thin and the holes of the honeycomb-like trabecular bone are enlarged. As your bones weaken, they become prone to fracture.

Like skin, bones are living, growing tissue. Throughout life old bone is removed (resorption) and new bone is laid down (formation). Special cells called osteoclasts dissolve bone tissue, while other cells called osteoblasts fill the cavities with new bone. This process is called remodeling and takes about four to eight months to complete.

Both cortical and trabecular bone are found throughout the body, but their proportions vary. Your spinal vertebrae and the ends of long bones in your arms and legs contain more trabecular bone. Because loss is more rapid in trabecular bone, osteoporosis tends to affect the hip, spine and wrist.

When you are young, you add new bone to your skeleton faster than old bone is removed. Starting around age eighteen, you reach your peak bone mass or your maximum bone density. Once peak mass is achieved, you will slowly start to lose bone and your body will no longer manufacture quite enough new bone to replace it. The denser your bones are before this process begins, the better your bone strength will be in later years.

After menopause, women begin to lose trabecular bone at a faster rate. This loss is due to falling estrogen levels and will continue for seven to ten years. Hormone replacement therapy can help counteract it. By age sixty-five, both men and women tend to lose cortical and trabecular bone at the same slow rate.

Who's at Risk?

Women—especially Caucasian and Asian women—are about four times more likely than men to develop osteoporosis. They have less bone mass than men to begin with, and their bone loss accelerates at menopause. In addition, women simply live longer than men. The government estimates that half of women over age forty-five and 90 percent of women over age seventy have some degree of osteoporosis.

Is There an Osteoporosis Gene?
Although as much as 60 percent of our chance for developing strong bones comes from how we live, heredity is still a major player in bone health. In 1994, researchers discovered a gene that contains instructions for a crucial vitamin D receptor. We need the receptor so our bones can use vitamin D to absorb calcium. If a version of this gene turns out to be a reliable marker for osteoporosis, women still in their teens will be able to take a blood test to assess their risk and begin preventive action decades before bone loss actually begins.

Osteoporosis causes about 250,000 hip fractures each year, and they occur three times more often in women than in men. Lean women who lose as little as 5 percent of their body weight after age fifty double their chance of hip fracture, as do women of average body mass who lose 10 percent of their body weight after age fifty. Researchers speculate that this link may be due to some combination of decreased muscle mass, less available estrogen from fat cells, less gravitational force on bone, and loss of natural hip padding. Most of these hip fractures cause some kind of permanent disability and 20 percent actually result in death.

Spinal fractures are also common in women over age fifty. Sometimes these fractures are painless, but they also can result in severe pain and disfigurement as the spine literally collapses on itself.

You are at even greater risk for osteoporosis if there is a history of the disease in your family. Heredity plays a role in your potential peak bone mass, determining just how strong your bones *can* become. Genes also determine the shape of your bones. Asian women, for example, have only about half the hip fractures of Caucasian women, even though both groups lose bone at about the same rate as they age. Researchers attribute the lower incidence of fracture to Asians' shorter hip axis, which is stronger and requires less bone density. Caucasians typically have a longer, weaker hip axis. Ironically, it is better nutrition in the preteen years that probably caused the height gain leading to a lengthened hip axis in Caucasian women.

Early menopause—before age forty-five—is another risk factor. The earlier your menopause, the more years you are without estrogen's protective effect on your bones. If you go through a natural menopause, you will lose estrogen gradually. If your ovaries are surgically removed, however, you will experience a sudden loss of estrogen.

What Can You Change?

Researchers compare bone health to a three-legged stool. To prevent bone loss, you need all three legs—estrogen, exercise and a well-balanced diet containing calcium.

We've looked at hormone replacement therapy earlier in this chapter and will consider it again in chapter 3. Estrogen reduces the rapid bone loss of the early menopausal years and has some ability to rebuild bone. If you decide to take estrogen, keep in mind that it doesn't promote strength, balance or muscle mass—all of which can help to improve your risk of falling and suffering a fracture. Those benefits come with exercise, the second leg of the stool.

Weight-bearing exercise, in which you carry your own weight—as in walking, running or stair climbing—is important in childhood when bones are being built. Once you've reached your peak bone mass, exercise helps keep bones strong. Studies have shown that postmenopausal women who exercise with weights twice a week can preserve bone density, become stronger and have greater balance than their sedentary counterparts. Strong back muscles can prevent the spinal compression fractures that lead to loss in height and stooped posture in osteoporosis victims.

Testing for Bone Density

The National Osteoporosis Foundation says that the best way to determine if you have even the earliest stages of bone loss from osteoporosis is to have a bone density test. You should have your bone density measured if you experienced early menopause, if you have had amenorrhea (a cessation of menstruation due to an eating disorder or too much exercise) or if you have a family history of osteoporosis.

If you've had a bone fracture that occurred due to very little trauma—like breaking a rib while coughing, you should consider a bone density test. And if you are debating starting hormone replacement therapy, you might want to have a density measurement done first to see how strong your bones are. Certain drugs, including thyroid hormones and steroids, can lead to osteoporosis. If you have taken medications like these, talk to your physician about bone density testing.

Bone density tests are safe, noninvasive and painless, and have become more available in recent years. After a bone test and a physical examination, your physician can assess your future risk for fracture and prescribe a course of treatment, if needed. After treatment begins, follow-up bone density tests should be done on the same machine or the same brand and model. Your doctor also might use blood and urine tests to monitor your progress.

There are several types of measurement devices available, and more in the pipeline. Most use a very low level of radiation. Dual-energy X-ray absorptiometry—DXA or DEXA—is the preferred method because it has the best resolution and uses only one-twentieth the radiation of a chest X ray. A DXA scan, which takes about five to fifteen minutes, measures bone density in the spine, hip and/or wrist, which are the most common sites for osteoporosis fracture. An "aged-matched" reading then compares your bone density to what is expected in someone your age, size and gender. A second reading, "young-normal," compares your results to the estimated peak bone mass of a healthy young adult woman.

Nutrition, primarily calcium, is the third leg of the osteoporosis prevention stool. Calcium is the principal component of bone. Your body can't manufacture calcium, and without it, you can't build bone mass. When a growing girl doesn't get enough calcium, her body will distribute what it does get among all her bones. Her growth won't be stunted, but her bones will be thin and weak. That's why more and more physicians are beginning to understand that osteoporosis is really a *pediatric* disease that manifests itself in later years.

One of the best ways to protect against osteoporosis-related fractures is to achieve the highest peak bone mass possible within the limits of your unique genetic programming. Researchers are learning that different bones peak at different times. The skull, for example, continues to increase in density through life. But the hip probably peaks in late adolescence and the vertebrae in the mid- to-late twenties.

Studies continue to show that a high-calcium diet is critical to building and sustaining bone mass all during the life cycle from childhood through the postmenopausal years. The only time calcium cannot substantially influence bone health is immediately after menopause. The approximate 15 percent of bone loss that occurs in the years just after menopause is largely a result of decreased estrogen. A postmenopausal woman has a greater need for calcium because without estrogen she not only doesn't absorb as much calcium but also secretes more than she used to in her urine.

In some situations, the current recommended daily allowance (RDA) for calcium may actually be too low. For example, in 1994, the National Institutes of Health recommended that post-menopausal women not taking estrogen boost their calcium intake to 1,500 milligrams daily. Researchers are continuing to explore how much calcium is needed to reach peak bone mass. The government has not mandated fortifying any foods with calcium because we are not sure how much calcium may be too much. For now, 2,000 milligrams is advised as a daily upper limit but new recommendations are being considered.

Recommended versus Optimal Calcium Intake for
Women (Milligrams Daily)*

Age/Situation	NIH Recommendation	Current RDA
Birth–1	400–600	400–600
Age 1–5	800	800
Age 6–10	800–1,200	1,200
Age 11–24	1,200–1,500	1,200
Age 25–49	1,000	800
Postmenopause	1,000–1,500	800
Pregnancy/lactation	1,200–1,400	1,200

*New recommendations are expected in late 1997.

The best source of calcium is dairy products. Unfortunately many teenagers and young women think that dairy foods are fattening. But researchers who study adolescent girls' eating habits have demonstrated that diary products like milk and yogurt can be added to the diet without weight gain, especially when these foods are lower-fat versions and are used to replace high-fat or empty-calorie foods like sugary snacks and soft drinks.

There are a few osteoporosis drugs that are especially useful for women who don't want to or can't take hormone replacement therapy. For example, the hormone calcitonin, available as a nasal spray, slows down bone breakdown. Alendronate, marketed as Fosamax, protects bone from being broken down and in tests on postmenopausal women, also appears to *build* high-quality bone. Both of these medications, as well as estrogen, work more effectively when combined with at least 1,000 milligrams of calcium daily. Another potential treatment, slow-release sodium fluoride, also may be more effective when supplemented with calcium citrate.

There's no doubt that calcium is a critical player in bone health, and we'll talk a lot more about how and why to add calcium to your diet, including what you need to know about supplements, in chapter 6. The way your body uses calcium and its interplay with other nutrients is an excellent example of why total diet is so important. For example, if you don't get enough vitamin D in your diet, and many older people do not, your body will have a harder time absorbing calcium. If you eat a lot of sodium or protein, your body may excrete more calcium than you can afford to lose. A woman who doesn't consume much sodium or protein may need as little as 400 milligrams of calcium a day. But if her intakes of both these nutrients are high, she may need 2,000 milligrams of calcium a day to offset urinary loss.

You may have heard that caffeine also affects calcium loss. This is another one of those controversial areas. A tablespoon or two of milk is enough to offset the effect of one cup of coffee. To be smart and cautious, limit your coffee to just a few cups a day.

Points to Remember

To maintain healthy bones:

◆ **Consider hormone replacement therapy if appropriate.**
◆ **Increase your exercise and include weight-bearing exercise.**
◆ **Get enough calcium in your diet.**

A FINAL WORD

We've looked at the incidence, risk factors and consequences of five diseases that are especially devastating to women—breast cancer, heart disease, diabetes, obesity and osteoporosis. Clearly, each of these conditions has a strong link to nutrition in prevention as well as treatment. Research on the role of nutrition in women's health is one of the most exciting frontiers of medicine. Do we have all the answers? No, not yet. But there are certain things we do know now. Among them is the fact that we must consider the total person and total diet over a lifetime. Good nutrition at any stage in life has an impact on disease risk and, consequently, on the quality of life women enjoy today and tomorrow.

CHAPTER 3

The Stages of a Woman's Life

As I began to write this chapter, the lyrics from one of my favorite songs kept running through my mind. It is from the Broadway musical *Barnum* and is called "The Colors of My Life." Part of it goes like this:

> *The colors of my life are softer than a breeze,*
> *The silver gray of eiderdown,*
> *The dappled green of trees.*
> *The amber of a wheat field,*
> *The hazel of a seed,*
> *The crystal of a raindrop are all I'll ever need....*

The stages of life we are looking at in this chapter are very much the colors of a woman's life. From puberty through menopause and beyond, women follow a path proscribed by the ups and downs of hormones like estrogen, but colored by unique life experience. We are learning that regardless of the path our hormones carve out for us, we are still responsible for making personal choices that affect our health and well-being. Nutrition is one of those choices.

Thanks to the women's health movement, the medical and scientific communities are finally beginning to recognize women's unique health needs. As a result of this new attention, we are learning more and more about the complex interplay of elements like hormones, nutrition and exercise that adds up to total health over a lifetime. In this chapter, we look at the basic nutritional needs of women at various stages of life. Check your life stage to see if you are doing all you can to ensure a healthy future. If you have a daughter or granddaughter, or if you are caring for an elderly friend or relative, you'll also find some information you might want to share.

ADOLESCENCE

Of all the advances made in women's health over the past decade or so, one of the most far-reaching is our growing understanding of just how important a healthy adolescence is to a healthy future. Like infancy, the teenage years are a time of significant growth and of extraordinary nutritional needs.

If you've spent time with adolescent boys and girls you know the three-part teen credo: Eat junk. Be cool. Live forever. But as adults, we've learned that life is not that simple.

An adolescent's passage into womanhood is marked by an increasing level of estrogen leading to menarche—the onset of the menstrual cycle. Teenage girls experience a growth spurt between ages ten and thirteen. (Boys catch up about two years later.) The growth spurt in height peaks about six to twelve months before menarche. The weight spurt usually peaks with menarche. Nutritional needs during these early teen years have less to do with chronological age and more to do with where an adolescent is in terms of this physical maturation process. Girls usually need the most calories in the year before menarche. But once her menstrual cycle starts, a teenager's nutrient needs will be more like those of an adult.

It's important for us to recognize that each girl is unique in the timing of her passage to womanhood. If you want to be sure your daughter gets off on the right course, the first step is to pay attention to how her nutrient needs change over time. During their "period of maximum growth," as it is officially called, teens add about 15 percent to 20 percent of their final adult height and 50 percent of their adult weight. Boys' skeletal growth occurs over a longer period than girls', and girls tend to deposit more body fat versus boys' muscle mass. Girls do not reach menarche until they have about 17 percent of total body weight as fat. This is why overweight teens often start their menstrual cycle at an earlier age, whereas lean athletic types begin later.

By age eighteen, one-third of a girl's weight is likely to be body fat. Unlike boys, girls keep most of the fat they put on in their teens into adulthood. And because lean body mass is more metabolically active, teenage boys typically burn more calories for energy than do girls.

An Investment in the Future

Good nutrition in adolescence is important not only to achieve full growth potential, but also to protect future health. But it's hard to convince someone who thinks she is immortal to look ahead to the possibility of chronic illness like heart disease, diabetes and osteoporosis. But looking ahead is essential for a lifetime of good health. And it is never too early to start.

Osteoporosis. There are two ways to prevent osteoporosis. One is to reduce the rate of bone loss after menopause. The other is to increase peak bone mass early in life (see chapter 2). We used to think that this crippling disease was inevitable in old age. But we've learned two important things: Osteoporosis is not inevitable and it is not a disease of old age. It is a pediatric disease. We now know that getting enough calcium during the teen years is critical to osteoporosis prevention (see Top Teen Minerals, page 62). Bone health is so important to future well-being that many schools now include some basic information on osteoporosis in their standard curriculum.

You have probably read articles extolling the virtues of weight-bearing exercise for building bone mass in *older* women. Well, it's just as critical for adolescent girls. The media hasn't caught up with the research, but judging from all the activity on bone health and adolescence in the scientific community, I'm certain it won't be long before the word gets out. In the meantime, all of us who have a teenage girl in our lives must work even harder to teach her how important exercise is to her well-being.

Heart Disease. Like osteoporosis, heart disease manifests itself later in life but may begin much earlier (see chapter 2). Autopsy studies show that early coronary atherosclerosis (arteries blocked by plaque) often begins in adolescence. We know that high blood cholesterol tends to run in families both because of genetics and a shared lifestyle. We also know that children with high cholesterol levels are more likely than the general population to have elevated levels as adults, too.

The government's recommended cholesterol levels for children and adolescents don't differentiate between girls and boys. But research on adults has shown us that one cholesterol level doesn't fit all (see chapter 4). Low HDL cholesterol, for example, is a stronger risk factor for heart disease in adult women than in men. Researchers are investigating how healthy cholesterol levels in young girls may differ from those in young boys. In the meantime, the best guidelines are:

Recommended Cholesterol Levels in Children* and Adolescents

	Desirable	Borderline /High Risk	High Risk
Total Cholesterol	below 170	170–199	200 and above
LDL Cholesterol	below 110	110–129	130 and above
HDL Cholesterol	35 and above		

*over age 2

For heart health, all children (over age two) and adolescents should follow the same healthy low-fat diet recommended for adults: 30 percent or less of calories from fat, including no more than 10 percent of calories from saturated fat; and less than 300 milligrams per day of cholesterol. And even though you may be holding down the fat, remember that teenagers still need energy (calories) and a wide variety of nutrients for proper growth. For both children and adolescents, extreme fat and calorie restriction is not recommended.

Following a heart-healthy diet not only helps prevent heart disease in later life, it also helps develop healthy eating habits that last a lifetime. Learning how to make smart food decisions early is also important for lifelong weight management.

Obesity. Adolescent obesity is an increasing problem with lasting repercussions—both physical and psychological. A chronic disease in its own right, obesity also is a risk factor for heart disease, diabetes and certain cancers (see chapter 2). Researchers cite lack of physical activity as a major contributor to obesity among teens. One study found a link between the prevalence of adolescent obesity and the number of hours watching television.

Statistics show that girls are at greater risk for obesity than boys. One out of five teenage girls is overweight, and the trend is on an upswing. A third of all obese women (compared to only 10 percent of obese men) were obese in early adolescence. Most men shed their extra teenage pounds; most women don't.

During a teenage girl's growth spurt, her body naturally produces fat. It's part of getting ready to bear children. But all the changes her body is undergoing can frighten a young girl. Survey after survey shows that many, if not most, teenage girls don't like their bodies. Seventy percent of girls diet between ages fourteen and twenty-one—whether they need to or not. Some of these so-called diets actually lead to weight gain. Sadly, even girls as young as eight can develop a distorted body image.

What is a healthy weight during adolescence? There is no precise answer. It depends upon a number of variables such as age, height and degree of sexual maturity. There's still a lot we don't know about obesity, especially in teenagers. It's a good idea not to embark on a weight-loss plan without first consulting a doctor or nutrition professional. Rather than prescribing weight loss for a moderately overweight teen, some doctors and nutrition professionals will suggest that she try to maintain her weight and let her height "catch up."

Unfortunately, worry about their weight and guilt about what they eat are constant companions for many teenage girls. But restricting calories is dangerous because so many nutrients are essential to growth and disease prevention during these critical growth years. This is the time when some young girls will turn to smoking to try to control their weight (see sidebar on page 60). Smoking accelerates metabolism and decreases appetite, but it's a sad and dangerous irony that the number-one and number-two causes of preventable disease and health—smoking and obesity—seem to cancel each other out. Medical experts say you'd have to gain 100 to 150 pounds over your ideal weight to equal the health risks of smoking. But in a society that idolizes being thin, when it comes to quitting smoking versus going up even one dress size, cigarettes often are the unfortunate choice.

Smoking: Don't Get Me Started!

Everyone knows that smoking is unhealthy, even if some choose to ignore the facts. Each year, more than 400,000 Americans die from tobacco-related illnesses such as lung cancer, heart disease and emphysema. The sad truth is that a half billion of the people alive today will eventually be killed by tobacco.

What is most frightening is that smoking is essentially a youth problem. Some 3,000 children—median age: twelve—start smoking each day. In a 1995 survey, nearly one in five eighth-graders, one in four tenth-graders and one in three twelfth-graders said they had smoked in the past month. The problem is especially acute among Caucasian teenage girls. Surveys show that most teenagers know that smoking is dangerous. They cite three reasons for pursuing the risky behavior anyway: Their friends do it. They're curious. It's "cool."

Smoking is unhealthy for both sexes, but women seem to have an even greater vulnerability. Since 1987, more American women have died of lung cancer than breast cancer, which, for more than forty years, had been the major cause of cancer death in women. Smoking also is an important risk factor for osteoporosis—almost exclusively a disease of women—because it interferes with the circulating estrogen that keeps bones strong. Chronic smokers also experience an earlier menopause, which means more years of bone loss due to lowered estrogen.

Research shows that smoking is also a major cause of heart disease among young and middle-aged women—especially those who are already at higher risk due to obesity, family history, hypertension, high cholesterol or diabetes.

An obsession with body image also can lead to life-threatening anorexia, bulimia or binge eating (see chapter 5). About eight million Americans—the vast majority of them female—suffer from eating disorders, and most of these people say their illness began before age twenty. We don't understand exactly what causes eating disorders. Researchers speculate that an imbalance of brain chemicals may be involved. Psychologists are exploring the link between eating disorders and self-esteem.

The physically active are not immune. Adolescent and young adult female athletes are at risk for a trio of related conditions called the female athlete triad—disordered eating, amenorrhea (the absence of three to six consecutive menstrual periods) and osteoporosis. Each one of these disorders is cause for concern; when combined, they can be deadly. Young women often believe that a diet with little or no fat is best for athletic performance. But the truth is that a certain amount of dietary fat is necessary to provide essential fatty acids and fat-soluble vitamins. Dietary fat is a concentrated form of energy that can be consumed in sensible amounts especially by athletes like runners, who have high calorie needs.

Unfortunately, low self-esteem, poor body image and depression go hand in hand for many young girls. Studies have shown that nine- to fourteen-year-olds are most vulnerable to losing their self-confidence. On television, in magazines, in the movies, young women are bombarded with the idea that being slim—even dangerously so—is beautiful and that extra weight is ugly. As a parent, be careful not to overemphasize your child's appearance. Ask yourself if your own body image and approach to dieting may be creating a dangerous environment for your daughter.

Talk About It!

Now that we are learning how important adolescent health is to lifelong health, we can look forward to more research on what it takes to build physical as well as emotional strength in teenage girls. Ongoing studies will help us develop more effective prevention strategies. In the meantime, nagging your teenagers—girls or boys—to eat right works no better today than it did in the past. It would be nice if we all could enjoy family meals together on a regular basis, but the reality is that busy lives often get in the way.

Today's teens are often left on their own to shop and cook—or to grab food on the run. From a nutrition standpoint, this autonomy doesn't have to be a bad thing. For example, if your daughter is going to be responsible for some of her own meals, she needs to know why and how to make smart food choices. Try to have an ongoing give-and-take conversation about making healthy food choices. Discuss what both of you are learning about new food products, food preparation and time-saving techniques. Make sure she knows that fortified cereal makes a good snack. Explain why and how a small fast-food hamburger—with lettuce and tomato, not bacon and cheese—can be a good choice for lunch. By talking, you both might learn something!

Most important, try to teach by example. Put the emphasis on what you can eat, not what you can't. Adolescents need good role models in many areas—including how to lay the foundation for a healthy future. And remember, teens don't want to give up their favorite foods any more than you do! The lesson of lifelong value is learning how to balance what you eat for enjoyment and good health.

Talk to your daughter as she approaches puberty. Tell her what to expect—how her body will change, how she might feel, what she will need to grow physically strong and emotionally resilient. Explain why healthy eating and exercise are important to her future. And look for ways to bolster her self-esteem. The more she cares about herself and her future, the more likely she is to invest in her good health.

Top Teen Minerals

Three minerals are especially important during the adolescent years, but that doesn't mean that *total* diet isn't important, too. Teens won't get enough calcium, iron and zinc—plus the energy and protein they need to grow—without eating a variety of nutrient-dense foods.

◆ **Calcium:** About 99 percent of calcium in the body is found in the bones and teeth. Because almost half of the adult skeleton forms during adolescence, teens—especially girls—need plenty of calcium (1,500 milligrams per day). Symptoms of calcium deficiency aren't likely to appear until much later in life. Getting enough calcium during the teen years helps girls fulfill their peak bone mass potential. The more bone mass a girl builds, the better off she will be as bone is lost later in life and osteoporosis becomes a threat.

Ironically, just when they need calcium the most, young girls tend to consume less. Teenage girls shy away from milk and dairy products, the richest sources of calcium, because they perceive these foods as fattening. As a result, most young girls are likely not to get the calcium they need. But recent studies show that girls can include dairy products in their everyday diet without gaining weight. Substituting yogurt for high-calorie, high-fat snacks and milk for high-calorie soft drinks are two steps in the right direction.

◆ **Iron:** Anemia can strike during infancy and adolescence—times when the body is building trillions of new red blood cells to carry oxygen and nutrients to a growing body. Teenage girls who diet and those who have heavy menstrual bleeding are at risk for developing iron-deficiency anemia. Symptoms include fatigue, dizziness, headache and irritability. Girls who are not yet menstruating require 12.5 milligrams of iron daily. After menarche the requirement jumps to 18 milligrams daily. Poultry, lean meats, legumes, green vegetables and iron-fortified cereal are good sources of iron. If her physician believes a young girl is at risk for anemia—perhaps because she is a vegetarian or a serious athlete—he or she may prescribe an iron supplement.

◆ **Zinc:** Essential for protein synthesis and growth, zinc is also particularly important for sexual maturation. For teenage girls the recommended daily intake is 12 milligrams. Good sources are poultry, lean meats, dairy products, legumes and whole grains. Chances are good that if a teen is getting enough protein, she is getting enough zinc as well.

For more on these minerals, see chapter 4.

Points to Remember

For teen health:

- ◆ **Protect future health with good nutrition during adolescence.**
- ◆ **Get enough calcium to build peak bone mass.**
- ◆ **Enjoy a low-fat diet to help prevent future heart disease.**
- ◆ **Recognize that obesity is a serious problem for some teens.**
- ◆ **Be aware that low self-esteem, poor body image and depression go hand in hand for some girls.**

THE CHILDBEARING YEARS

Fertility

One out of five couples in the United States is infertile. Up to age thirty-four, women's fertility rates are fairly constant. Between ages thirty-five and thirty-nine, infertility becomes more common. Infertility rates increase again after age forty. Many of the causes for infertility are not yet known. We do know, however, that some infertility is related to nutrition and usually can be corrected.

Like many of the health issues with a link to nutrition, fertility is a matter of balance—especially when it comes to body weight. Being too thin or too heavy can interfere with ovulation; not ovulating is one of the most common reasons for infertility in women. The connection between body weight and ovulation is estrogen. The ovaries produce estrogen and so do fat cells. If your body fat is low, you will produce less estrogen. If your body fat is high, you'll produce more. Either way, you can throw your reproductive cycle out of balance.

Let's look at the effects of being overweight first. Studies have shown that obese women (with a BMI of 27 or greater) have a significantly higher risk of being anovulatory, meaning they do not ovulate and consequently cannot become pregnant. Although we know estrogen is involved, we don't exactly know

---

Are You "on the Pill"?

If you use birth control pills over an extended time, you may be affecting your body's ability to absorb and use certain nutrients. Deficiencies in vitamin B_6, for example, may trigger some of the mood-related side effects of the pill, such as depression, anxiety and insomnia. Vitamin B_6 is necessary for the brain to produce serotonin, a chemical that regulates pain, mood and some eating behaviors (see chapter 4).

If you are deficient in vitamin B_6 before you start taking birth control pills, the situation will only get worse. Often all that is needed to relieve the mood problems associated with the pill is some more vitamin B_6 in your diet to counteract the pill-induced deficiency. (Chicken, pork, fish, bananas, spinach and potatoes are good sources of vitamin B_6. Whole grains, nuts and legumes also contain B_6.) In some cases, a supplement might be recommended. Check with your physician or a nutrition professional.

Birth control pills are also associated with weight gain, increased appetite and reduced absorption of folic acid. A folic acid deficiency early in pregnancy can lead to birth defects like spina bifida. Making sure your folic acid level is optimal is one reason your doctor will advise you to wait six months to conceive after you stop the pill.

---

how all the pieces of the puzzle—estrogen, weight, diet and ovulation—fit together. For now, though, it's safe to say that if you are having trouble conceiving and are not at a healthy weight, your first step should be to change your food and exercise habits. If you take off the extra weight now, you'll enjoy a healthier pregnancy, too.

If you are too thin, you are likely to suffer from amenorrhea, which means your menstrual cycle is stalled and you are not ovulating. Once again, the link is estrogen. Infertility related to low body fat may account for 25 percent to 30 percent of all cases of infertility in U.S. women. If you are an athlete, if you suffer from anorexia nervosa or if you are simply underweight, your body fat may fall below the level needed to maintain a normal menstrual cycle.

There is some evidence that having had an eating disorder earlier in life can affect fertility later. If researchers are able to confirm and explain this connection, it will give us yet another reason to emphasize the importance of nutrition and health in the teenage years when young girls are so vulnerable to anorexia and bulimia.

Fertility can also be affected by the balance of certain micronutrients in your diet. For example, all vitamins are important for good health, but if you are trying to become pregnant, you should pay special attention to B_6, C, D and E.

◆ **Vitamin B_6:** Several studies show that deficiencies of vitamin B_6 can lead to hormone irregularities that affect fertility.
◆ **Vitamin C:** Balance is the key word with this vitamin. Megadoses of vitamin C can reduce fertility.
◆ **Vitamin D:** Because it aids in calcium absorption, vitamin D is critical to bone health. A deficiency in vitamin D could result in a weak pelvis, making it difficult for a woman to carry a full-term, healthy-weight baby.

◆ **Vitamin E:** Although vitamin E has no direct effect on human fertility, it does influence prostaglandins, which are hormonelike substances that play an important role in reproduction.

Deficiencies in the minerals magnesium, potassium and zinc are also associated with infertility. You may hear that certain vitamins or minerals taken in megadoses enhance fertility. If you are trying to become pregnant, this is not the time to experiment. Follow the advice of your doctor or a nutrition professional. There is still a lot we don't know about how nutrients interact, especially when we tamper with the synergy of a balanced diet. You are in a vulnerable position. Once you do conceive, you'll want your baby to grow in a safe, healthy environment for the next nine months.

For more about vitamins and minerals, see chapter 4.

Points to Remember

For health during the childbearing years:

- ◆ **Maintain a healthy weight.**
- ◆ **Keep vitamins and minerals in balance.**
- ◆ **Never experiment with megadoses of nutrients.**

Pregnancy

You might be surprised to learn that of the approximately four million U.S. women who give birth each year, six in ten experience some health problems during pregnancy or delivery—and half of these problems are major. That's why it's important to go into pregnancy as fit as you can be and to start prenatal care as soon as possible. Nutrition is one of the best tools to ensure a healthy and safe pregnancy.

A normal pregnancy lasts about thirty-eight to forty weeks. A significant portion of a baby's organ development occurs in the first three months (first trimester). During the next six months or so,

Rx for Morning Sickness

That queasy feeling in the morning is one of the first signs of pregnancy. About half of all pregnant women experience morning sickness during the first three months.

Morning sickness actually can strike any time of day and can last indefinitely. It's most common, though, when your stomach is empty. Vitamin B_6 has been used to treat nausea and vomiting during pregnancy, but there is no research to back up its effectiveness. And taking one of the B vitamins alone can upset the balance of the other vitamins at work in your body.

Here are some tips to ease the symptoms of morning sickness:

- ◆ Eat small, frequent meals through the day.
- ◆ If you tend to be sick in the morning, nibble on plain crackers, popcorn, dry cereal or vanilla wafers before you even get out of bed. This will help remove excess acid from your stomach.
- ◆ Get up slowly to avoid aggravating nausea.
- ◆ Drink liquids slowly. Don't drink beverages or soups with meals, but be sure to get enough liquid between meals, especially if you are vomiting.
- ◆ Eat more starches like bread, pasta and potatoes.
- ◆ Avoid foods and cooking aromas that have brought on nausea in the past—for example, coffee or fried foods.

In about 2 percent of pregnant women, morning sickness can become so severe that it interferes with lifestyle, leads to dehydration and affects the body's ability to absorb vital nutrients. If nausea is severe or persists for more than three months, or if you are losing weight, be sure to consult your doctor.

the baby's vital organs continue to develop, physical features are defined, and he or she grows and puts on fat. Meanwhile, the mother's body is changing dramatically, too.

Women's bodies are built to adapt to the state of pregnancy. For example, blood volume doubles and the chambers of the heart enlarge to pump more efficiently. The heart beats more rapidly and the heart muscle itself becomes stronger. Veins become larger to handle the extra blood flow. As much as 20 percent of the blood a pregnant woman's heart pumps goes to the uterus.

A pregnant woman's respiratory rate increases and her bladder expands to hold twice as much urine. The kidneys work overtime and the pelvis begins to soften. The stomach makes less gastric acid and the immune system adjusts to allow for the presence of antigens it doesn't recognize—those from the baby's father. During the first half of pregnancy, a woman releases more insulin to help regulate glucose.

Food to Grow On. While all these changes are occurring, it's important to make food choices that will help the process, not hinder it. Let's start by looking at calories. What's enough? How many are too many?

The total "cost" of pregnancy is about 80,000 calories above and beyond normal needs. That works out to an increase of about 285 calories a day over a nine-month period—or a total of about 2,500 calories a day for the average woman. And when you're pregnant, every calorie has to count toward providing nutrients for you and your baby. There is no room for empty calories. If you are underweight going into pregnancy or if you are very physically active, you'll need more calories. If you're overweight you'll need fewer.

The Vitamin-Mineral Connection

Pregnancy is not the time to skimp on any vitamins or minerals. You need to meet your baby's needs as well as your own. Here are a few micronutrients that are especially important.

◆ **Calcium:** If your diet doesn't provide enough calcium, your baby will take what he or she needs to build a skeleton from your bones, putting you at greater risk for osteoporosis later in life. Some studies also show that proper calcium levels help prevent high blood pressure and toxemia. You'll also need to keep your calcium intake high if you breast-feed. The recommended daily intake of calcium is 1,500 milligrams for pregnant and breast-feeding women. Milk and dairy products are the best sources of calcium.

◆ **Folic acid:** Because it plays such a critical role in cell development, pregnant women need more folic acid (a B vitamin) than usual. Research shows that taking folic acid before pregnancy and during early pregnancy can reduce the risk of low birth weight and neural tube defects like spina bifida. All women of childbearing age are urged to consume 400 micrograms of folic acid daily (twice the normal intake). To help you meet this goal, in 1998 food processors will begin fortifying flour and other grain products with folic acid. You also need folic acid if you are breast-feeding. Your baby can deplete your stores, impairing your ability to build red blood cells and leaving you anemic.

◆ **Iron:** Iron is used to build red blood cells. Over the course of pregnancy, you absorb an extra 1,000 milligrams of iron, and your daily iron requirement doubles from 15 milligrams to 30 milligrams. Your body needs more iron because your blood volume increases by about 50 percent and your baby needs iron to build his or her own blood cells. If you enter pregnancy with low iron stores, you may become anemic. Your need for iron will increase as your pregnancy progresses. During the last months, the demand for iron is especially high because your baby is building his or her own iron reserves. The amount of iron in breast milk is low, so babies need to store some extra iron to use during the first few months after birth. Poultry, lean meats, legumes and green vegetables are good sources.

◆ **Vitamin D:** You always need this vitamin for the absorption of calcium—and you require twice as much if you're pregnant or breast-feeding. The recommended daily intake is 10 micrograms or 400 international units. Milk is fortified with vitamin D.

Although it's possible to meet the pregnancy and lactation requirements for most vitamins and minerals with a balanced diet, your doctor will probably recommend a daily supplement, which should contain the following micronutrients.

Nutrient	Amount milligrams (mg)/ micrograms (mcg)
Calcium	250 mg
Copper	2 mg
Folic Acid	400 mcg
Iron	30 mg
Vitamin B_6	2 mg
Vitamin B_{12}	2 mcg
Vitamin C	50 mg
Vitamin D	5 mcg
Zinc	15 mg

To promote absorption of these nutrients, supplements should be taken between meals or at bedtime. Remember that if taken in large doses, vitamins can be toxic. We'll talk about vitamins and minerals again in chapter 4.

If your diet is too low in calories—fewer than 1,800 calories per day—chances are your baby won't get the protein he/she needs to grow. The RDA for protein during pregnancy is sixty grams. Most pregnant women get at least this much protein if they are eating enough calories.

The primary source of calories for pregnant women should be carbohydrates in fruits, vegetables and whole grains, In general, everyone, including pregnant women, should get more than half of their calories from carbohydrates. Restricting carbohydrates when you are pregnant can be dangerous. Your baby's nervous system needs the glucose produced from carbohydrates to develop properly. Some glucose can be made from protein, but that cuts into protein's main function of tissue building. And when glucose is made from fat reserves, a toxic byproduct develops called ketones, which could be harmful to your baby.

Fiber, which is a type of carbohydrate, is important during pregnancy because it helps prevent constipation, which is a common problem, especially in the last months of pregnancy. Although there's no specific guideline for fiber in the diet during pregnancy, you'll want to eat plenty of fruits, vegetables, legumes and whole-grains for their many nutritional advantages—including fiber.

By now you've heard at least a million times that fat should be limited to 30 percent or less of calories. This guideline is a good one to follow during pregnancy, but fat should not be overly restricted. Your baby needs a fat called linoleic acid for the development of brain cells and the central nervous system. Since linoleic acid is not produced by your baby, you need to provide it. Safflower, sunflower, corn and soybean oils are good sources.

We used to think that sodium should be restricted during pregnancy because it supposedly contributed to hypertension. A number of studies have shown that the hypertension characteristic of pregnancy is not related to salt. You may need to restrict sodium, however, if you have the kind of hypertension that is affected by salt intake. Your doctor should give you the guidance you need.

This is an important issue because more salt is needed by a woman during pregnancy than at any other time in her life. Cutting back on salt can interfere with the expansion of the mother's blood volume, which is critical to supplying the baby with nutrients. But you probably don't need to worry about getting enough sodium. Between what is naturally found in food, what's added in processing, and what's used in cooking and at the table, all of us get more than enough.

Water is also an important nutrient that is often overlooked during pregnancy. You need water because of increases in your blood volume and to help maintain your body temperature. You also need more water to help dilute your baby's waste products so they can be excreted in your urine. In general, we're well advised to drink eight glasses of water a day. If you're pregnant, increase your intake to ten glasses.

Finally, a word on alcohol. Over the past twenty years or so, the thinking about alcohol and pregnancy has changed. Today's advice is very simple: No amount of alcohol is considered safe during pregnancy. Some experts maintain that just one drink a day can lead to fetal alcohol syndrome (FAS). Babies born with FAS are abnormally small at birth and don't have the same amount of brain tissue. These children may be severely mentally retarded, and many have heart defects and other abnormal internal organs.

Why Weight? Throughout this book, I stress that dieting is a bad idea. Let me emphasize here that if you are pregnant, dieting is a *really* bad idea. Nowhere is the concept of healthy weight—and healthy eating as a way to get there—more important than in pregnancy and while you are breast-feeding.

If you don't gain enough weight during pregnancy, your baby may have a low birth weight (under 5 1/2 pounds), which puts him/her at greater risk for disease and even death during the first month of life. You also need to store fat if you are planning to breast-feed. On the other hand, if you gain too much weight during pregnancy you won't have a bigger baby, but you will store that weight as fat. Getting back to a prepregnancy healthy weight will be harder. There is some evidence that gaining too much weight can also lead to complications during delivery.

A general guideline for weight gain is twenty-five to thirty-five pounds. If you are underweight when you become pregnant, your range is slightly higher: twenty-eight to forty pounds. Overweight women are advised to gain about fifteen to twenty-five pounds. One reason to try to reach a healthy weight before pregnancy is that overweight women who become pregnant may be at higher risk for having babies with neural tube defects like spina bifida—even if they take the 400 micrograms of folic acid daily that is recommended to prevent such birth defects.

If you are five feet two inches or shorter, aim for the lower end of the weight range. Pregnant women under eighteen should gain at the higher end of the range because they themselves are still growing. Should you double the weight range if you're having twins? No, just ten extra pounds (thirty-five to forty-five) will do.

If twenty-five to thirty-five pounds sounds like a lot of weight to you, take a look at how that weight is distributed in a mother who gives birth to a seven- or eight-pound baby.

	Approximate Weight Gain (lbs.)
Baby	7–8
Placenta	1–2
Amniotic fluid	2
Mother	
Breasts/uterus	3
Increased blood volume	3
Body fat	5 or more
Increased muscle tissue and fluid	4–7
Total	25 pounds minimum

Your pattern of weight gain is also important. In the first few months of pregnancy, you probably will gain very little weight— maybe as little as two to four pounds. After that, you should gain about one pound a week. If you are gaining weight too fast, talk to a nutrition professional about how to modify your diet without depriving your baby of the nutrients needed for growth and the nutrients you need for optimal health.

Researchers speculate that weight gain during pregnancy may be connected to obesity later in life. Even women who limit their weight gain to the recommended range tend to retain some weight after delivery. Of course, the more children you have, the more this extra weight adds up. Nevertheless, pregnant women must not be discouraged from gaining enough because they are worried about their weight slowly creeping up after every baby. More research is needed in this area, to protect both growing babies and their mothers.

Weight loss after pregnancy should be gradual. Often, it takes nine months to a year to achieve prepregnancy weight, depending on age, activity level, how much weight was gained and whether or not the mother is breast-feeding.

Through the Ages. Older women and younger women have some special nutrition needs and concerns during pregnancy. If you become pregnant after age thirty-five—and many women today are doing just that—your metabolism has already started to slow down, so you need fewer calories to maintain a healthy weight. But you need just as many nutrients as a younger pregnant woman.

Women over age forty have a slightly higher risk of developing gestational diabetes, which increases the chance for high blood pressure and toxemia (a dangerous condition characterized by general swelling, excess protein in the urine and hypertension). Gestational diabetes usually doesn't occur until the end of the second trimester. Women with this complication tend to have big babies and sometimes must have a cesarean delivery. They also are likely to develop overt diabetes later in life.

The American Diabetes Association recommends that *all* pregnant women be tested for diabetes in the twenty-fourth to twenty-eighth week of pregnancy. Gestational diabetes can be treated with diet and exercise, while still meeting nutrient needs and recommended weight guidelines. You can still have a very healthy baby if you are diagnosed with gestational diabetes. But consult with a nutrition professional immediately so that you can develop an individual eating and exercise plan to control what can become, if left untreated, a very dangerous complication.

Pregnant adolescents also face some special health and nutrition challenges. The younger the girl, the greater the risk for a premature or low-birth-weight baby. Adolescents are also at greater risk for toxemia and anemia. The pregnant teenager has to consume enough calories and nutrients for her baby's development and for her own growth.

Bone health is particularly important in the teen years. Since peak bone mass is building until at least age twenty-five and sometimes beyond, calcium is a critical nutrient for young adults. A pregnant teenage girl and her baby will compete for the calcium and vitamins necessary to build bones. And while some adolescents have a problem with gaining too much weight, others gain too little—often because they are worried about their body image. Pregnant adolescents ages eleven to fourteen need about 2,700 calories daily; pregnant teens ages fifteen to eighteen require about 2,400 calories each day.

Breast-feeding: Your Choice. As far as your body is concerned, breast-feeding is part of the total experience of pregnancy. During the nine months your baby is growing, your body is getting ready to produce breast milk.

Choosing whether or not to breast-feed and for how long are very personal decisions. Health experts recommend breast-feeding because it benefits both mother and baby. Breast milk is custom-made to meet the baby's energy and development needs, and the composition of the milk changes as the infant's needs evolve. Antibodies and other special components in breast milk protect babies from respiratory and intestinal infections. Breast-feeding offers health benefits to mothers as well. Women who breast-feed may lower their risk for premenopausal breast cancer and ovarian cancer.

Some of the extra fat you store away during pregnancy is mobilized later to make breast milk. But breast-feeding is by no means a quick weight-loss plan. Most of the energy needed to make milk comes from the calories you eat after your baby is born. You need about 650 extra calories a day to breast-feed. Ideally, 500 of these nutrient-dense calories come from food added to your normal intake. The other 150 calories come from your body's own fat stores. Most women have stored 4.5 to 6.5 pounds of fat, which is enough to supply 100 to 150 calories a day over a six-month period.

Breast-feeding, as an extension of pregnancy, is not the time to diet. If your daily calorie intake drops below 1,800, you probably won't get the nutrients you need and you'll endanger your milk supply. Breast-feeding will increase your own need for calcium, magnesium, zinc, vitamins B_{12}, D and B_6, and folic acid. Your normal diet will probably provide enough protein, especially if you are eating low-fat dairy products for a calcium boost. If you took a prenatal vitamin-mineral supplement, your doctor may have you continue taking it while you breast-feed.

Points to Remember

For health during pregnancy:

- ◆ **Maintain a healthy weight during pregnancy.**
- ◆ **Take a prenatal supplement.**
- ◆ **Drink lots of water.**
- ◆ **Don't skimp on calcium.**

Premenstrual Syndrome

It's the subject of a lot of jokes, but when *you* have premenstrual syndrome, it's not so funny. Few women totally escape PMS, but for many, symptoms are minor. Others, however, are incapacitated by premenstrual symptoms for several days or even a couple of weeks every month.

PMS is not a disease in the classic sense. You can't be tested for it, symptoms can vary from month to month and from woman to woman, and medical experts really don't know what causes it. The term *premenstrual syndrome* was coined in 1931, and PMS first appeared in the American Psychiatric Association (APA) reference manual in 1985 as Late Luteal Phase Dysphoric Disorder (LLPDD), primarily a mood disturbance. In 1994, the APA recognized the most severe form of PMS as a type of major depression and labeled it Premenstrual Dysphoric Disorder (PMDD).

This move has been controversial. Some people believe it promotes the idea that all premenstrual women are mentally ill and supports the stereotype that women are victims of their biology. If you think this is a nonissue—think again. We definitely don't want to return to the time not so long ago when all women's health issues were linked only to our reproductive organs. Consequently, women must be very clear about the complexities of PMS. Historically, myths about menstrual impairment are given more attention in times when women are making social advances—in education, business and politics. Yes, PMS symptoms are themselves a reality, but we must be careful that they are not used to explain away the realities and the uniqueness of women's complicated, often stressful lives.

As many as 200 different symptoms have been reported in association with PMS. Common physical symptoms include breast tenderness, a craving for salt and sweets, abdominal bloating and headaches. Common psychological symptoms are irritability, anxiety, depression, low self-esteem and hostility.

Although women of all ages can have symptoms of PMS, the

condition is most common in women over age thirty. It often becomes more pronounced after childbirth or after cessation of birth control pills. PMS typically worsens with age and in later years may be confused with the symptoms of menopause.

Diagnosing PMS. PMS tends to be overdiagnosed. Sometimes women label mood swings as PMS when, in fact, they are natural emotional cycles—plain and simple mood swings. Pelvic infections, diabetes and depression can be misdiagnosed as PMS. If you answer yes to the following three questions, what you are experiencing is likely to be PMS:

◆ Do your symptoms occur between ovulation and the time your period starts, go away in about two days and stay away for about two weeks?

◆ Has this pattern repeated itself for at least three consecutive menstrual cycles, and have you and your doctor ruled out other physical or psychological causes?

◆ Are your symptoms frequent and severe enough to interfere with your life?

It seems obvious to blame PMS on the rise and fall of estrogen and progesterone that occur during the luteal phase, or last two weeks of the menstrual cycle. When you consider the fact that PMS symptoms don't occur before puberty or after menopause (unless you're taking hormone replacement therapy), it is clear that somehow hormones are involved.

Some researchers speculate, however, that while PMS may coincide with the menstrual cycle, it may be unrelated to it. For example, symptoms may be related to circadian rhythm (body clock). Other investigators think PMS may be related to hormonal changes that occur during the *first* two weeks of the menstrual cycle, rather than the last two weeks.

The "feel-good" brain chemical serotonin and natural pain-relievers called endorphins may provide yet another link to PMS.

Both substances increase with higher levels of estrogen and progesterone. But when levels of these reproductive hormones abruptly fall off about a week or so before your period starts, some brain chemicals decrease as well. The food cravings associated with PMS are likely an effect of this changing brain chemistry (see chapter 5).

PMS Symptoms

As many as 200 different PMS symptoms have been documented. They involve water retention, behavioral changes, nervous system reactions, negative emotions, pain and other physiological manifestations. Some of these symptoms include:

Physiological	*Psychological*
Acne	Anxiety
Backache	Confusion
Bloating	Depression
Constipation	Forgetfulness
Diarrhea	Hostility
Dizziness	Insomnia
Fatigue	Irritability
Food cravings (salts and sweets)	Low self-esteem
Headache	Panic attacks
Irregular heartbeat	Paranoia
Joint and muscle pain	Violent behavior
Nausea	
Rashes	
Poor motor coordination	
Weight gain	

Estrogen and progesterone also affect blood sugar, which tends to be low in the last two weeks of the menstrual cycle. Low blood sugar can cause PMS-like symptoms of dizziness, headache, irritability, anxiety and fatigue. PMS symptoms also may be related to stress. What we don't know is which comes first—the stress or the PMS.

Looking for Relief. Dietary treatments for PMS are a popular topic in women's and health magazines. Let's review some of the most frequent recommendations.

Vitamin B_6 and magnesium deficiencies have been implicated in PMS because these nutrients affect brain chemicals like serotonin and dopamine, which induces relaxation and mental alertness. Some women with PMS who have taken B_6 and magnesium supplements report relief from their symptoms, but this may be just a placebo effect. Vitamin B_6 is especially controversial because when taken alone, it can deplete other B vitamins and in large doses, it can cause nerve damage.

Boosting your calcium intake is another popular PMS treatment. Calcium is also thought to play a role in regulating brain chemicals that affect mood and in reducing water retention. We already know that calcium is vital in fighting osteoporosis. If you are getting enough calcium for good bone health, you're getting enough for PMS relief as well. Meanwhile, studies to document the effect of calcium on PMS continue.

Vitamin E also might help relieve PMS symptoms, but we need to see results of more research before we can be certain there is a link here. You also might have heard that evening primrose oil is a good antidote for PMS. So far, however, research has not confirmed a link between evening primrose oil and PMS relief.

Phytoestrogens, which are compounds found in foods like soy, also may relieve some PMS symptoms. These weak plant estrogens can attach to the body's estrogen receptors and may deliver the benefits of estrogen without any negative effects. We don't yet know what amount of phytoestrogen is needed for PMS relief and we don't know how they interact with other hormones. This is a new frontier in nutrition research that you can expect to hear a lot about in the future.

If you have PMS, are there foods you should avoid? In the past, we have recommended cutting down on sodium to help alleviate water retention and swelling. Now there is evidence that the hormone progesterone, which rises during the last two weeks of the menstrual cycle, may act as a diuretic that causes you to excrete a lot of sodium in your urine. Cravings for salt may result. Unless you gain five to seven pounds prior to your period, you probably don't need to restrict your salt beyond the general recommended daily intake of 2,400 milligrams. If your doctor suggests you use a diuretic, replace the potassium and magnesium you are likely to lose through excess urine by eating bananas, apricots, potatoes and leafy greens.

Caffeine's role in PMS is unclear. Although it can act as a natural diuretic if you are bloated from excess water, some research indicates that it may aggravate the tenderness caused by fibrocystic breast disease (the cyclical "lumpy breasts" condition that affects more than half of all women). Caffeine has also been implicated in bone loss leading to osteoporosis. Try to limit your caffeine to the equivalent of one cup of coffee a day. It's also wise to limit your alcohol intake during the premenstrual phase of your cycle. Because it is a depressant, alcohol can worsen the mood swings that are typical of PMS.

Finally, exercise is often recommended as a treatment for PMS. In addition to all its other positive effects—like strengthening bone and muscle and building heart and lung capacity—exercise helps relieve PMS anxiety and depression by stimulating the release of brain endorphins, natural mood elevators that make you feel good after exercising. Right before your period starts, your endorphin level is particularly low.

Breaking a sweat during a workout cuts water retention and reduces bloating and puffiness. But you don't have to sweat to reap the benefits. Even moderate exercise reduces PMS symptoms. Another exercise bonus is that it helps keep your weight stable if you tend to eat more right before your period.

The bottom line on using a megadose of any kind of supplement or food to relieve PMS symptoms is this: We're not exactly sure what really works because we're not sure what really causes PMS. With the possible exception of calcium, which some women may need to take in supplement form for osteoporosis prevention, the safest approach is to get the nutrients you need from a well-balanced diet. There's no harm, however, in trying to relieve PMS symptoms by cutting back on salt, caffeine and alcohol. One or more of these approaches might work for you. And don't forget exercise. It may not cure all your PMS symptoms, but it has so many other benefits that it is definitely worth a try.

Points to Remember

For coping with PMS:

- ◆ **Eat a balanced diet rather than megadoses of any nutrient.**
- ◆ **Experiment with limiting salt, caffeine and alcohol.**
- ◆ **Increase your exercise.**

GROWING OLDER . . . AND BETTER

Menopause

Before we begin, let me emphasize an important fact: Menopause is *not* a disease—any more than puberty is a disease (although some of us with teenagers may have wondered). Unfortunately, Western culture has medicalized menopause, when in fact it is a normal biological event.

In some West African, South American and Native American societies, postmenopausal women are revered. They are elevated to positions of authority in the family and looked to as spiritual leaders and healers. If you review Western history, however, you'll see a pattern of treating menopausal women as old crones past their prime. Menopause has been seen not as a beginning but as an end.

It's Normal. What happens at menopause is normal—for women. What happens to men and their testosterone as they age is normal—for men. Place either gender in the other's health paradigm and, of course, you'll see "abnormalities." And that's exactly what has happened with women and menopause. We have spent a lot of years in a medical paradigm that used men's health as the norm. This is one reason our culture looks at menopause as an illness. The fact that we don't know very much about menopause, and that much of what we do know is based on the experience of women with problems, only adds to the perception that menopause is a disease rather than a normal passage of life.

Menopause is garnering more attention lately because we are realizing that women do in fact have unique health needs. And there are more women approaching menopause. On average, menopause occurs around age fifty (see sidebar). More than 40 million American women are over age fifty now. That's greater than a third of the female population. By the year 2000, more than 21 million women will reach age fifty at the rate of 1.3 million a year. And with the potential life span now pushing eighty, many women can expect to live almost a third of their lives after menopause.

Menopause and puberty are at opposite ends of a hormonal continuum. Just as estrogen and progesterone slowly rise in a preteen girl, they slowly ebb in an older adult woman. Unpleasant short-term symptoms can arise at either end of this mirror-image process. Teenage girls may experience acne, weight gain and moodiness; older women may experience hot flashes, weight gain and moodiness.

Pre-, Peri- and Post-: Understanding the Menopause Markers

Have you ever noticed that as soon as women reach age thirty-five or so, they often begin to refer to themselves in one of three ways: premenopausal, menopausal or postmenopausal? Women who are really in the know include "perimenopausal," too. What do all these terms really mean?

◆ **Premenopausal:** You're still having regular periods and have not experienced any changes in menstrual flow.

◆ **Perimenopausal:** You've been experiencing changes or irregularities in your menstrual flow for a year or so that can't be attributed to other causes. You may have an occasional hot flash or mood swing. Perimenopause usually starts in the mid-forties as your ovaries gradually produce less estrogen and progesterone. It lasts four to six years. Women in perimenopause often say they are "going through menopause."

◆ **Menopausal:** Your actual time of menopause is determined retrospectively. Technically speaking, menopause is the day twelve months after your ovaries have released their final egg—that is, a year after your last period. Heredity plays a significant role in when you will reach menopause; the average age is fifty-one.

◆ **Postmenopausal:** You are postmenopausal when you have not had a period for more than a year and can't attribute this to anything other than menopause.

Women who have both ovaries removed experience surgical menopause, which is very different from natural menopause. Unlike the gradual loss of estrogen that comes with natural menopause, surgical menopause triggers a dramatic drop in estrogen.

Some of the symptoms of menopause are very apparent (see sidebar), and they are the ones that tend to disappear after the body gets used to a new level of hormones. Physiologic changes that occur after menopause are not as obvious, at least not for a number of years. These changes, having to do with heart and bone health, are intimately tied to estrogen.

Signs You Can't Miss

Some women will have none of the short-term symptoms of menopause. If you are like most women, however, you will experience a few—especially hot flashes. Most of these disturbances will go away when your body adjusts to its new hormone levels.

The classic symptoms of menopause listed here are related to what is called vasomotor instability, which occurs when a hormone imbalance causes your normal temperature-regulating mechanisms to overreact and affect your blood vessels.

- Hot flashes and night sweats
- Vaginal dryness
- Heart palpitations
- Insomnia
- Tingling feeling in the skin
- Off and on numbness, especially in the fingers
- Joint and muscle pain
- Dizziness
- Shortness of breath
- Dry eyes and dry mouth

Short-Term Changes. Hot flashes and night sweats occur when the body's internal temperature gauge is somehow confused. We suspect lowered estrogen has something to do with this thermostat but don't yet know the exact connection. Almost

60 percent of American women experience sudden feelings of intense heat, flushing and profuse sweating. But in Eastern cultures where women eat a lot of foods like soy that are rich in phytoestrogens, hot flashes are almost unknown. It may be that these weak plant estrogens are strong enough to keep the "estrogen set point" from wavering. It is likely, though, that phytoestrogens are not acting alone but are interacting with other nutrients and perhaps other hormones.

Vitamin E (30 milligrams to 300 milligrams) may ease hot flashes, but there are no definitive studies to support this approach. Check with your doctor before you take large amounts of this nutrient.

Depression and moodiness have also been associated with menopause and, unfortunately, have provided a lot of fodder for jokes at the expense of women. Right up there with the fact that menopause is not a disease is the fact that menopausal women are not crazy! The "menopausal madness" theory has no basis and is simply a leftover from another era.

Recent studies have shown that menopause causes neither depression nor psychosis. When a menopausal woman is diagnosed with a clinical mental illness like depression, she probably had the illness before menopause became a factor. Many women actually greet menopause with relief.

A lot of how you react to menopause will depend on your life at the time—how happy and fulfilled you feel. Some menopausal women are moody and out of sorts from time to time. In addition to the stress of everyday family life and work life, this moodiness may result from lack of sleep due to night sweats. We also know that estrogen reacts with certain brain chemicals. A lack of estrogen may result in lower levels of serotonin, a neurotransmitter that affects feelings and sleep patterns and triggers food cravings. A drop in serotonin also may help explain why you have a premenstrual craving for sweets. Low serotonin levels can be boosted with carbohydrates, but aim for the nutrient-rich complex carbohydrates of whole grains more often than you go for an empty-calorie sugar fix.

Menopause is also associated with weight gain—even among women who never had a problem with weight before. We know that women often do gain weight at this time in their lives, but it probably has more to do with age than anything else. Metabolism—the rate at which you burn calories—slows with age, primarily because you begin to lose energy-burning muscle. Most of us—men and women—need to eat fewer calories and exercise more to build muscle and keep weight stable.

Long-Term Effects. Among the hidden effects of menopause are its long-term impact on bone health, heart health and breast health.

Osteoporosis: After reaching your peak bone mass—somewhere around age twenty-five—you will gradually begin to lose bone, increasing your risk for osteoporosis and bone fractures of the hip and wrist. This bone loss also weakens the spine, which may begin to collapse, slowly taking inches off your height and causing a dowager's hump (see chapter 2).

At menopause, when estrogen levels start to fall rapidly, you will experience a substantial loss of bone. There's no getting around this fact. The earlier your menopause, the greater your risk for osteoporosis. What makes a big difference at this point is your peak bone mass—that is, how much bone you were able to build before bone loss began. Your peak bone mass *potential* is genetic. Whether or not you fulfill that potential is up to you. As I pointed out earlier, a lot depends on your calcium intake when you were younger. Several years after menopause, your bone health will once again depend on calcium plus exercise to build strength and balance (see chapter 6). And if you are taking an osteoporosis drug, it will work best in tandem with calcium. As you'll see when we discuss hormone replacement therapy (HRT), estrogen is also critical.

While calcium is your number-one defense in the nutritional management of osteoporosis, it is by no means the only important nutrient. Vitamin D helps your body absorb calcium. And tipping the balance in the opposite direction, excess protein and sodium in the diet will lead to excreting too much calcium in your urine. Bone health is a perfect example of why total diet is important and why good nutrition is a lifetime concern. Calcium is a key nutrient in osteoporosis prevention and treatment, but it doesn't act in isolation. The need for calcium starts in childhood, and it's just as important at fifteen as it is at fifty and beyond. See chapter 6 for more about calcium.

Heart Disease: Until you reach menopause, you'll have a much lower risk of heart disease than a man does. But after your estrogen levels drop off, all bets are off. Heart disease is the number-one cause of death among postmenopausal women (see chapter 2).

Although we don't understand exactly how, lowered estrogen at menopause causes women's protective HDL cholesterol to drop and dangerous triglyceride levels to rise. This combination heightens the risk for heart disease. Although hormone replacement therapy can reverse this trend, diet, exercise and lifestyle (no smoking!) still play a critical role in the prevention of heart disease.

Breast Cancer: Breast cancer is also more common in postmenopausal women (see chapter 2). Late menopause is one of the risk factors for breast cancer because estrogen can foster the growth of breast tumors. There is also some evidence that HRT may heighten the risk for breast cancer.

Researchers suspect that a high-fat diet may contribute to breast cancer, but so far studies have yielded conflicting results. We do know that a diet high in fruits, vegetables and grains and low in fat has many health benefits. I believe the chances are excellent that we will soon prove breast cancer prevention to be one more of those benefits. I think we will also confirm that nutrition during the teen years—when breasts are forming—has an impact on the future risk of breast cancer. Once again, total diet and a lifetime of healthy eating will emerge as a front-line defense against disease—in this case, the disease women fear most.

Points to Remember

For menopause:

◆ Recognize that menopause is not a disease, but rather a normal life passage.

◆ Get enough calcium and vitamin D for bone health.

◆ Monitor your HDL cholesterol and triglyceride levels to help prevent heart disease.

◆ Enjoy a low-fat diet.

◆ Consider hormone replacement therapy, if appropriate.

Hormone Replacement Therapy

Remember the Clairol ad that used to ask, "Does she, or doesn't she?"? You might hear the same question posed today—but now it's about hormones, not hair color. And with twenty-one million baby boom women approaching menopause over the next decade, we're going to hear a lot more about hormone replacement therapy (HRT) in the years to come.

Sometimes you will see the acronym ERT, which stands for estrogen replacement therapy. Back in the 1970s, ERT was hailed as a fountain of youth for women. It helped keep bones strong and relieved menopausal symptoms like hot flashes. Then in the early 80s, researchers discovered that women who took estrogen had a much greater risk for endometrial cancer. It looked as though the glory days of hormone replacement would be short-lived. For women who still had their uteruses, estrogen replacement was just too dangerous.

In the early 1980s, scientists discovered that combining estrogen with progestin (a synthetic form of progesterone) eliminated the risk of endometrial cancer. This combination approach is called HRT—or hormone replacement therapy. Recent research has shown that HRT not only relieves short-term symptoms of menopause like hot flashes, vaginal dryness and moodiness, but also offers the same *long-term* heart and bone protection as the "unopposed" estrogen of ERT.

Pros and Cons. Although we don't yet know if HRT actually *reduces* heart disease—no study has lasted long enough to confirm that potential effect—we do know that HRT significantly lowers heart disease risk by raising protective HDL cholesterol and lowering dangerous LDL cholesterol. HRT also lowers levels of the protein fibrinogen, a blood-clotting factor predictive of heart attack and stroke. Women with high fibrinogen levels have twice the risk of heart attack as women with low fibrinogen.

At one time, researchers thought that these results might be influenced by what is called a "confounding factor"—in this case, that women who take HRT typically are at lower risk already because they tend to be more health-conscious and have better access to medical care. But subsequent research confirmed that the heart-healthy benefits of HRT are not confined to this select group of women. Studies show that HRT can lower heart disease risk by 12 percent to 25 percent in postmenopausal women. Considering that heart disease is the number-one killer of American women (see chapter 2), this is an important breakthrough.

As far as bone health is concerned, it has long been known that estrogen increases the absorption of calcium and encourages bone formation. One theory is that estrogen keeps bone-building osteoblasts and bone-thinning osteoclasts in balance (see chapter 2). Research shows that combined hormone replacement theory (estrogen plus progestin) is just as effective in preserving bone health as estrogen alone.

HRT also may reduce the risk of colon cancer, the third leading cancer killer of women. Studies found that women who took estrogen alone or combined estrogen-progestin therapy for more than ten years cut their colon cancer risk by nearly half. Some scientists speculate that the production of certain bile acids involved in colon cancer may be reduced by estrogen. Others believe that estrogen acts directly on the lining of the colon to suppress tumor growth. Clarifying the link between colon cancer and HRT will continue to be a challenging area for research.

You also may have seen reports in the media about estrogen's potential role in preventing and treating Alzheimer's disease. This is important news because two-thirds of Alzheimer's victims are women. Estrogen is thought to improve blood flow in the brain and to stimulate nerve cell growth in the regions of the brain affected by Alzheimer's. Researchers believe that the reduction in risk is about 5 percent for every year on estrogen therapy. And among those afflicted with Alzheimer's, estrogen seems linked to a milder impairment. Again, the link between estrogen replacement therapy and Alzheimer's is a subject of ongoing research.

There has been some controversy over whether or not hormone replacement therapy causes weight gain. Current thinking is that HRT is not associated with the weight gain commonly seen in postmenopausal women.

Despite all this good news about HRT, there is a potential downside: HRT may promote breast cancer. The proliferation of breast cells caused by constant exposure to estrogen can trigger cancer (see chapter 2). Taken for five years or less, estrogen does not appear to increase breast cancer. Unfortunately, though, it is the long-term use of HRT that fights heart disease and osteoporosis, and your risk of developing either of these diseases far outweighs your risk of breast cancer. Research also suggests that, for women at risk for breast cancer, alcohol and HRT don't mix. Studies show that women on HRT who drink as little as one drink a day significantly increase their amount of circulating estrogen. If you have had breast cancer or if either your mother or sister has had breast cancer, your doctor will probably advise against HRT (see sidebar).

The HRT Frontier. If you are not able or don't want to take traditional HRT, you may be a candidate for one of the emerging alternative forms of hormone therapy. For example, if you are seeking relief from menopausal symptoms—and not necessarily long-term heart- and bone-health benefits—you might want to talk

HRT: Should You or Shouldn't You?

Despite documented long-term benefits, only 25 percent of American women ages forty-five to sixty-four are on HRT. Potential side effects and the annoyance of taking daily medication cause about a fifth of women who start HRT to quit within nine months. And most women quit after three years or less. Is HRT right for you?

If your answer is yes to these questions, HRT may be a good choice for you:

- ◆ Do you have a family history of premature heart disease?
- ◆ Do you have high LDL cholesterol?
- ◆ Do you have a family history of osteoporosis?
- ◆ Are you having severe hot flashes or other menopausal symptoms?
- ◆ Are you willing to put up with the potential PMS-like side effects of some HRT regimens?
- ◆ Are you willing to take medication for many years?
  If your answer is yes to this question, think twice about HRT.
- ◆ Do you have a family history or personal history of breast cancer?

to your doctor about estriol, which is now available in a low-dose skin patch. Your body actually produces three types of estrogen: two potent forms, estradiol and estrone, and a weaker form call estriol, which is at its highest level during pregnancy. You can take a plant-derived estriol without progestin because it does not increase your risk for endometrial cancer and, in a low dose, probably does not contribute to breast cancer either.

You may have heard of tamoxifen, a drug used in breast cancer therapy. Tamoxifen is actually an antiestrogen. It was once thought that all antiestrogens did was block estrogen's cancer-promoting effect on breast tissue. Scientists subsequently discovered that antiestrogens also have some of the positive heart-health and bone-health effects of estrogen. Drugs like tamoxifen are in the vanguard of research on hormone therapy. The ultimate goal is to mimic estrogen's positive activities in certain cells and limit its negative activities in others.

The National Institutes of Health Postmenopausal Estrogen/ Progestin Interventions Trial (PEPI) has yielded much of what we already know about the effects of HRT. In 1993, the Women's Health Initiative began a ten-year study of the impact of HRT, low-fat diet, calcium and exercise in preventing cancer, heart disease and osteoporosis. Results from this massive study, some of which will be available in the next several years, not only will put HRT into the context of total health but also will tell us how long it is safe to take HRT, how long it should be taken for optimal benefits, and how the need for HRT might change with age and with nutritional health.

If you are considering HRT, discuss the risks and benefits with your doctor. There are at least fifteen different estrogen preparations on the U.S. market plus about five estrogen-progestin combinations. Making an informed decision about HRT isn't easy. But no decision you make needs to be permanent. There's a lot of new information about HRT on the horizon.

Points to Remember

About hormone replacement therapy:

- ◆ **Know your risks before starting HRT.**
- ◆ **Make an informed decision.**
- ◆ **Keep your eye on new developments in HRT.**

The Later Years

How old is old? As life spans increase, the definition of old changes as well. What was thought of as old in our grandparents' day is now regarded as middle-aged—or younger. Today, when we talk about seniors and older people, we usually mean those age sixty-five and over. When we talk about the elderly or oldest old, we're usually referring to people eighty-five and up.

Women in their forties responding to a survey by the Collagen Company said they believe old age doesn't begin until seventy-two—just a few years shy of women's life expectancy! As the first baby boomers start turning sixty-five in 2011, so-called old age is likely to have a decidedly younger twist. And due to the sheer numbers of people in the boomer generation, we'll probably begin to learn a lot more about the aging process. We will have a golden opportunity to learn more about women and age—an area that has been neglected for too long.

It's not surprising that there is a knowledge gap. To date, scientists have directed most of their detective work on aging to discovering cures for fatal diseases. Much less time and resources have been devoted to investigating how normal aging makes us vulnerable to disease and what we might do about it. In addition, as I explained in chapter 1, until recently, women were routinely excluded from medical research. The one investigation into aging, the Baltimore Longitudinal Study, which began in 1958 and continues today, didn't even include women until after 1978.

This omission is especially ironic when you consider that women typically outlive men by about seven years. Of the thirty-three million Americans age sixty-five and older, twenty million are women. By the year 2050, two-thirds of all Americans over age eighty-five will be women. This isn't a new phenomenon. Throughout history, women have had a longevity advantage. Mummified bodies dating as early as A.D. 500 show that even then women lived longer than men.

Scientists speculate that women may be hardier from conception. Although male fetuses outnumber female fetuses by almost 115 to 100, only slightly more male babies are born than female babies. By age thirty, the population ratio becomes just about even and from that point on, women become the majority.

Among the top-ten killer diseases, every one except diabetes kills significantly more men than women. Theories explaining this disparity in longevity range from the effects of stress to a genetic vulnerability based on the male XY chromosome. But most researchers believe it is related to estrogen and the wide-ranging protection it gives women.

The average human life span has crept up over the centuries from about 28 in colonial America to almost 50 at the turn of the century. Since 1900, male life expectancy has increased by 25 years, while 28.6 years have been added to female life expectancy. Better sanitation, antibiotics to control infectious disease and safer childbirth are largely responsible for this rise in longevity.

The next frontier is nutrition. Although good nutrition can't reverse the health status of the current generation of older people, it can contribute to improving their quality of life. As we learn more about what actually happens to the body as we age, we'll be able to identify how healthy eating over a lifetime contributes to longevity and vitality.

Weighing In on Aging. One of the areas researchers are continuing to investigate is the effect of weight on healthy aging. As you age, you need fewer calories to maintain a healthy weight because lean body mass decreases and your metabolism slows. But needing fewer calories doesn't mean you need fewer nutrients. Balancing calories, nutrients and exercise to maintain a healthy weight is a real challenge at any age. But if you are older and need to drop a few pounds, you'll be encouraged to know that people in their seventies actually are more successful at losing weight than people in their thirties.

Weighing too little as you get older can be just as much of a health risk as weighing too much. Carrying your own healthy body weight strengthens your bones, and weight provides protective padding that helps protect bones from breaking. If you are too thin, you may not have the nutrient reserves you need during an illness or after a surgery.

You may have read about research on rats showing that severely restricting calories, while keeping nutrient intake high, extends their life span. So far, no evidence indicates this approach will work for humans, too. In fact, an extremely low calorie diet may have a negative impact on the immune system, cause nutritional deficiencies (leading to osteoporosis or anemia, for example) and result in malnutrition. And severe calorie restriction just plain takes the fun out of eating! If you are already at a healthy weight, don't restrict your calories below what is recommended to maintain that weight. Many older adults need about 1,600 calories daily. If you need help determining your best weight, how to attain it and how to keep it, ask your physician for a referral to a nutrition professional.

Sometimes older people lose weight because they are depressed and have no interest in food. Studies show that depression affects as many as 40 percent of elderly Americans, and it's the most common cause of weight loss in nursing home patients. Depression can be caused by a number of factors, including deaths of spouses and friends, difficulty with the demands of everyday living, loss of independence and a diminished sense of purpose. It also may result from some illnesses and is a side effect of many medications. Depression must be taken very seriously because it is a life-threatening disease in its own right. If you yourself are depressed or if you are caring for an older person who seems to be depressed, talk to your physician immediately.

DHEA: Is It Medical Magic?

DHEA—dehydroepiandrosterone—has been billed as the superhormone that can slow the aging process, promote weight loss, prevent heart disease, prevent or alleviate Alzheimer's disease, and fight cancer, AIDS and lupus. It sounds like medical magic, but the truth is we know very little about how DHEA works in the body (other than that it is converted into other hormones like estrogen and testosterone). And we know even less about the potential long-term effects of taking DHEA supplements.

A chemical cousin of estrogen and testosterone, DHEA is a steroid hormone made from cholesterol by the adrenal glands. Early in life, your adrenals don't manufacture very much DHEA. Production really kicks in at about age six or seven and peaks during the mid twenties. DHEA levels begin to taper off around age thirty until by eighty, most people have only about a fifth of the DHEA they had fifty years earlier. DHEA levels also fall during illness, regardless of age. Only humans and other primates produce DHEA, and males tend to have higher levels than females.

The Food and Drug Administration banned over-the-counter sales of DHEA in the mid-1980s, when it was being marketed as a weight-loss aid. Since 1994, health food stores have been allowed to sell an alleged precursor to DHEA made from wild yams, but scientists say the body does not convert any plant steroid into DHEA. The hormone is available, however, as a drug, and some doctors are prescribing it for patients despite its potential risk.

Many of the experiments done with DHEA have been performed on rats and mice, and the findings are not necessarily applicable to humans. Studies on humans have produced mixed results and inconclusive findings. But we do know that taking DHEA can result in some far-reaching negative side effects for women, including growth of body or facial hair. In addition, some premenopausal women stop menstruating. DHEA can also decrease levels of HDL cholesterol in women, increasing the risk of heart disease. Researchers don't yet know the impact of DHEA on breast cancer.

Although some people taking DHEA report feeling energetic, invigorated and even "reborn," it will take years of additional research to uncover the real secrets of this mystery hormone. In the meantime, don't be fooled by all the hype. Just because something is "natural" doesn't mean it is safe. DHEA is a good example of this fact. When we disturb the balance of nature, there are always consequences. And when it comes to DHEA, too many of these consequences are still unknown.

Your Changing Nutrient Needs. Your body's need for certain nutrients may change over time.

Carbohydrates: The major job of carbohydrates is to provide energy. To give your body enough fuel to burn, about 50 percent to 60 percent of your total calories should come from carbohydrates. Fiber, which is found in foods like grains, vegetables and fruits, is important to help prevent constipation.

Fat: The need for dietary fat does not change with age. The body needs some fat in order to get essential fatty acids and enough fat-soluble vitamins. A diet low in saturated fat and dietary cholesterol is generally recommended to keep blood cholesterol at safe levels. Some research shows, however, that a low *total* cholesterol count may not be as important to heart health in people over age seventy. As with younger people, high HDL cholesterol may be protective against heart disease in the elderly, too. While physicians may not prescribe cholesterol-lowering drugs for people over seventy, it's a good idea to continue with a diet low in fat (30 percent of calories) and low in saturated fat (10 percent of calories). When you have fewer calories to enjoy, why use them up on high-calorie fat?

Protein: Because your body becomes less efficient at using protein, you need more of this nutrient as you get older. The fifty grams of protein generally recommended for younger adults is too low for the elderly. A lack of protein in the diet may result in depressed immune function, loss of muscle strength and poor wound healing. Older women need about sixty grams of protein daily. Some older people who have a difficult time getting enough protein add a liquid medical nutritional supplement to their diet.

Vitamins and Minerals: How your body uses certain vitamins and minerals also can be affected by age. Before you decide to take any type of supplement, review your current food intake with a nutrition professional who can help you determine which micronutrients may be missing from your regimen. Your need for a particular nutrient can vary based on your age, health and lifestyle.

Water: Dehydration is one of the most frequent causes of hospitalization of people over age sixty-five. As you get older, a lower percentage of your body weight will be fluid, your thirst sensation won't be as strong and your kidneys may not concentrate urine as they used to. Sometimes, a fear of incontinence or trouble getting to and from the bathroom will lead an elderly person to cut back on fluids. People who live alone are especially vulnerable, particularly when they have the flu or diarrhea. To safeguard against dehydration, be sure to drink at least six to eight cups of water or other fluids a day.

In chapter 4 we will take a more detailed look at vitamins and minerals and where they are found in food. In the meantime, here is a quick rundown of the micronutrients likely to be most important to you as you get older.

◆ **Antioxidant Vitamins:** A, C and E are antioxidant vitamins that work to diffuse damaging free radicals that are byproducts of normal metabolism and of various toxins in the environment. Immune cells are particularly sensitive to free radicals. Some scientists maintain that as cells die in the aging process, even more free radicals are formed. Thus, the older we get and the more free radicals we have, the more damaged our immune system can become. Free radicals have also been implicated in cataracts and in age-related macular degeneration, which is the leading cause of blindness in people over sixty-five.

In addition to acting as an antioxidant, vitamin C plays an important role in helping the body absorb iron. It is possible to get enough vitamin C from a well-balanced diet, but studies have shown that some elderly people are at risk for a deficiency, especially since the body doesn't store this vitamin.

Although older people may ingest less vitamin A, they seem to store it more efficiently than younger adults do. Vitamin E deficiencies are rare and not considered a risk for elderly people. There is some evidence that a high intake of vitamin E from food or supplements may lower your risk for heart disease, cancer and premature aging.

◆ **B Vitamins:** Folic acid lowers blood levels of a chemical called homocysteine, which is linked to heart attack and may be involved in stroke as well. Folic acid also helps in the manufacture of red blood cells, and a deficiency may lead to anemia. A deficiency in vitamin B_{12} also can result in anemia as well as in neurological problems like poor balance and impaired memory. A B_{12} deficiency may develop in older people because they become less able to absorb the nutrient. Some older adults may need more B_6 in their diets than the 1.6 milligrams needed daily by younger people. A vitamin B_6 deficiency can affect immunity.

◆ **Vitamin D:** Vitamin D is especially important to older women because it helps the body absorb and use calcium to retain bone. Older adults typically have lower levels of active vitamin D because they consume less from food. The body can manufacture vitamin D when the skin is exposed to sunlight, but many older people no longer spend sufficient time outdoors, and overexposure to sunlight can cause skin cancer.

◆ **Minerals:** Both calcium and phosphorous are critical to bone health in elderly women. The third player on the bone health team is vitamin D, which is necessary for calcium absorption. Because many elderly women cannot get enough of these micronutrients in their regular diet, your doctor may want you to take a supplement.

Iron is important for women of all ages. Iron absorption can be impaired if, as you grow older, your body secretes less gastric acid for digestion or if you take antacids. Diuretics, laxatives and antacids can affect your zinc level, resulting in a loss of taste and appetite and slow wound healing. Low zinc levels can also compromise the immune system.

What About Tomorrow?

Women are more likely than men to require long-term care. One reason is that they tend to live long enough to need it. But it's not just a matter of age. Even the "young" among older women (sixty-five plus) are more likely than men to have "activity of daily living" (ADL) limitations brought on by chronic conditions that limit mobility, such as arthritis and osteoporosis. They are also more likely to have heart disease and diabetes. Almost half of women over age eighty-five have problems managing daily tasks like eating and bathing; 65 percent have difficulty with at least one activity like preparing meals or shopping.

Aging women also face the very real prospect of less than adequate health care in general. For example, studies show that older women may not receive the same quality breast cancer treatment as younger women. Their treatment for heart disease and hypertension also may be less than optimal. If an older woman sees only a gynecologist, she may not be screened for diabetes or colon cancer. If she sees only an internist, she may not receive a pelvic exam, Pap smear or mammogram.

What can you—as an older woman or as a caregiver—do about this situation? First, you must do what you can to safeguard your own health and independence. Follow a healthy diet—like the one outlined in chapter 6—and be sure to exercise. You can't fight heredity but you can live up to your genetic potential. Considering that cardiovascular disease and cancer account for the majority of all deaths, doing what you can to reduce your risk for these diseases may add years to your life. You can also cut your risk for osteoporosis, which is both a crippler and a killer. Of course, there are no guarantees, but healthy eating and exercise won't hurt you and certainly will improve the quality of your life.

Second, demand high-quality preventive care and treatment from your health-care providers. Keep in mind that older women are more likely than older men to use outpatient services. As a result, women are an important part of the practices of primary-care physicians. Be your own advocate and ask for what you need. If possible, see a board-certified geriatrician or a doctor with at least some training in geriatrics.

Finally, get involved in making changes in the health-care system. Let your state and federal legislators know how important accessible, high-quality long-term care is for women. Recent elections have shown that women's votes swing elections, so use your clout!

Points to Remember

About growing older:

- ◆ **Maintain a healthy weight.**
- ◆ **Recognize your changing nutrition needs.**
- ◆ **Demand quality health care.**

CHAPTER 4

Your Nutrition Tool Kit

I've been a nutrition professional for twenty-five years, but I've been a lover of good food for much longer than that. I don't think food is about rules. I think it's about friends, family, memories, great flavors and good health. But since there is so much conflicting information these days, it's hard to know what to believe about food and health. I don't want to give you rules, but I do want to share some basic nutrition guidelines with you. I want you to build a foundation of facts so that no matter what new information or controversies arise, you'll be able to make informed and sensible decisions.

Currently, we know that more than forty different nutrients are needed in sufficient quantity and in the right proportion to prevent nutritional deficiencies or excesses that can affect your health. The macronutrients—fat, carbohydrate and protein—provide the calories we need for energy and, in the case of protein, the amino acids we need to build body tissues. The micronutrients—vitamins and minerals—are essential for a vast array of essential body processes.

But we don't eat nutrients. We eat food. And the fact is there are many ways to combine foods for a healthy diet. It's a matter of personal choice, and you don't have to be a nutrition scientist to figure out a plan that works for you.

Think of your body as a high-performance machine. Like any fine piece of equipment, your body runs more efficiently when you pay attention to the "owner's manual"—in this case, the Dietary Guidelines for Americans and the Food Guide Pyramid. The Dietary Guidelines explain how to eat to promote good health (see sidebar The Dietary Guidelines for Americans, below). The Food Guide Pyramid is like a blueprint for total diet (see illustration, page 108). It shows you how to turn the Dietary Guidelines into food choices. It guides you toward a variety of foods and helps you keep your diet balanced so you get all the nutrients you need. Finally, the food label—both the nutrition facts panel and the ingredient list—is the special tool you need to compare foods so you can make informed decisions (see illustration, page 113).

The Dietary Guidelines for Americans

- ◆ Eat a variety of foods.
- ◆ Balance the food you eat with physical activity; maintain or improve your weight.
- ◆ Choose a diet with plenty of grain products, vegetables and fruits.
- ◆ Choose a diet low in fat, saturated fat and cholesterol.
- ◆ Choose a diet moderate in sugars.
- ◆ Choose a diet moderate in salt and sodium.
- ◆ If you drink alcoholic beverages, do so in moderation.

THE DIETARY GUIDELINES

The Dietary Guidelines represent consensus among the nation's leading health and nutrition experts about the role of nutrition in maintaining health and minimizing the risk of major chronic diseases in the United States. The guidelines are general because they must apply to everyone over two years of age. All the country's major medical groups endorse the Dietary Guidelines. Some—like the American Heart Association and the American Cancer Society—also publish their own guidelines. These guidelines actually complement the Dietary Guidelines by providing similar messages as well as emphasizing the specific nutrition concerns of the sponsoring group.

The first Dietary Guidelines were published by the government in 1980 in response to a growing awareness of nutrition's relationship to a number of chronic diseases. The 1995 Dietary Guidelines are the fourth revision, and it is now law that the guidelines be reviewed every five years in light of new scientific findings.

Revisions in the most recent version of the Dietary Guidelines reflect evolving scientific knowledge as well as our changing attitudes toward health and food. For example, because so many people are now vegetarians or semivegetarians, the latest guidelines include a brief discussion of meatless eating and point out that some nutrients may be harder to get when all foods of animal origin are excluded from the diet. The latest guidelines also emphasize exercise more than earlier versions did, noting that increased physical activity is important not only for weight control but also for adequate immune function and overall good health. Earlier versions of the Dietary Guidelines included two sets of healthy weight ranges—one for younger and one for older adults. The 1995 edition maintains that health risks associated with excess weight are the same at any age and emphasizes the importance of weight maintenance throughout adulthood.

One of the most meaningful changes in the 1995 guidelines is that eating a lot of grains, fruits and vegetables is emphasized over choosing a diet low in fat. Previously, it was the other way around. This subtle change is especially important for two reasons: First, it's a *positive* approach to healthy eating—a *do* eat, not a *don't* eat. Second, although most people now know that a low-fat diet has many health benefits, many don't understand the importance of grains, fruits and vegetables—not to mention what a wide variety there is to explore, taste and enjoy.

Another subtle but meaningful change in the guidelines concerns sugar and salt. Previous editions zeroed in on both of these nutrients and strongly advised using them "only in moderation." The latest edition takes a broader perspective, suggesting we choose a *total diet* moderate in salt and sodium—in other words, keep your focus on the big picture. Remember, there are no "good" or "bad" foods.

(You can download a copy of the booklet *Nutrition and Your Health: Dietary Guidelines for Americans* from the U.S. Department of Agriculture Food and Nutrition Information Center Web site at http://www.nal.usda.gov/fnic.)

THE FOOD GUIDE PYRAMID

The U.S. Department of Agriculture and the Department of Health and Human Services introduced the Food Guide Pyramid in 1992. Although not mandated by law, periodic review of the pyramid is likely to go hand in hand with review of the Dietary Guidelines.

The Food Guide Pyramid turns the Dietary Guidelines into actual food choices by depicting the combination and the proportion of complete foods you need for a healthy diet. As a graphic representation of your total diet, it illustrates both variety and balance while focusing on reducing fat.

Each of the five food groups comprising the pyramid provides some, but not all, of the nutrients you need each day. Recommended daily servings are expressed in a range—for example, six to eleven servings from the grain group. Your number of recommended daily servings from each group depends on personal characteristics such as age, gender and level of physical activity. If you are fairly sedentary, you may need only about 1,600 total calories a day and, therefore, only six servings from the grain group. If you are very active, you may need as many as 2,800 calories each day and eleven servings from the grain group. Because the Food Guide Pyramid illustrates servings for a day's worth of food, you don't have to limit your planning to one meal at a time.

When planning your meals, work from the bottom of the pyramid up. The idea is that by the time you get to the tip of the pyramid—high-calorie fats, oils and sweets—you'll be choosing smaller amounts of food. You can pack a lot of variety into one salad with a couple of servings of pasta, an array of fruits and vegetables, perhaps a bit of cheese or some nuts or meat, herbs, and a light touch of salad dressing. Dishes like these that combine a number of dif-

Food Guide Pyramid
A Guide to Daily Food Choices

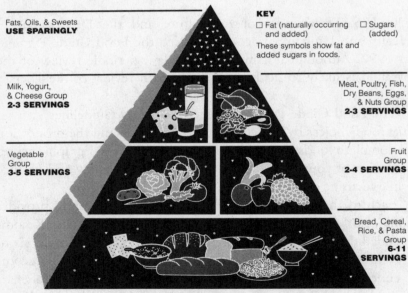

Fats, Oils, & Sweets
USE SPARINGLY

KEY
☐ Fat (naturally occurring and added)   ☐ Sugars (added)
These symbols show fat and added sugars in foods.

Milk, Yogurt, & Cheese Group
2-3 SERVINGS

Meat, Poultry, Fish, Dry Beans, Eggs, & Nuts Group
2-3 SERVINGS

Vegetable Group
3-5 SERVINGS

Fruit Group
2-4 SERVINGS

Bread, Cereal, Rice, & Pasta Group
6-11 SERVINGS

Source: U.S. Department of Agriculture/U.S. Department of Health and Human Services

ferent foods are common in our everyday diet, and it's easy to see how they can reflect the variety and balance the pyramid promotes.

What Is a Serving?

The Food Guide Pyramid suggests a range of servings for each food group. The right amount for you depends on your age, gender, body size and activity level. But after you know how *many* servings are recommended, you still need to know exactly how much food is in a serving. Here are some guidelines:

Food Group	Serving Size
Bread, Cereal, Rice and Pasta	1 slice bread; 1 English muffin; 1/2 bagel; 1 oz. ready-to-eat cereal; 1/2 cup cooked cereal, rice or pasta; 5–6 small crackers; 2 medium cookies
Vegetable	1 cup raw leafy greens, including endive, escarole, romaine, spinach or other salad greens; 1/2 cup cooked or chopped raw vegetables, including carrots, cauliflower, green beans, leeks and peppers; 3/4 cup vegetable juice; 1 medium tomato; 1 medium potato; 5 asparagus spears; 7–8 carrot sticks; 1 ear of corn on the cob
Fruit	1 medium apple, banana, orange or peach; 2 medium plums or tangerines; 1/3 cantaloupe; 1/8 honeydew melon; 15 small grapes; 1/2 cup cut-up raw, cooked or canned fruit; 3/4 cup fruit juice; 8 medium strawberries; 3/4 cup blueberries; 1/4 avocado

Milk, Yogurt and Cheese	1 cup milk or yogurt; 1 1/2 oz. natural cheese; 2 oz. processed cheese; 1/2 cup ice cream, ice milk or frozen yogurt
Meat, Poultry, Fish, Dry Beans, Eggs and Nuts	2–3 oz. cooked lean meat, poultry or fish; foods that count as 1 oz. of meat = 1/2 cup cooked dry beans, 1 egg, 2 tablespoons peanut butter, 1/3 cup nuts.

You may notice that some of these serving sizes don't match the serving sizes you find on food labels. For example, on a food label, two slices of bread comprise one serving, but in the pyramid one slice is one serving. Many health and nutrition groups fought for a standard pyramid and label serving sizes, but the wheels of bureaucracy can create inconsistency. Here is what I recommend: Use the serving sizes recommended in the pyramid as your guideline for planning a balanced diet. Use the food label to help you compare similar foods and make healthy choices.

Food Guide Pyramid
Sample Food Plan for a Day

The Food Guide Pyramid gives a daily range of servings for each food group. What's right for you depends on your daily calorie requirements, which are determined mostly by your age, gender and activity level.

The National Academy of Sciences has made some general recommendations for adults and teenagers based on national food consumption surveys: 1,600 calories a day is about right for many sedentary women and some older adults. Most children, teenage girls, active women and many sedentary men need 2,200 calories. Pregnant or breast-feeding women may need more. Teenage boys, many active men and some very active women need about 2,800 calories daily.

	Calories		
	1,600	*2,200*	*2,800*
Bread Group	6 servings	9 servings	11 servings
Fruit Group	2	3	4
Vegetable Group	3	4	5
Milk Group	2–3*	2–3*	2–3*
Meat Group	5 oz.	6 oz.	7 oz.
Total Fat Grams**	53	73	93

*Pregnant/breast-feeding women, teenagers and young adults to age twenty-four need three servings.
**Based on 30 percent of calories as recommended by the Dietary Guidelines.

Because you probably don't carry measuring spoons and a food scale with you, here are some handy ways to judge the serving size of a portion of food:

This much food . . .	*. . . is as big as:*
1/2 cup vegetables	Tennis ball
1 cup of lettuce	4 green leaves
1 medium potato	Computer mouse
1 medium whole fruit	Your fist
1 1/2 oz. of cheese	Three dominoes
3 oz. of meat, fish or chicken	Deck of cards, cassette tape or bar of soap

THE FOOD LABEL

In the 1980s, food companies realized that in addition to wanting convenience and good taste, consumers also wanted more healthful food choices. But as more manufacturers made health claims about their products, consumers seemed to become more confused. And because serving sizes were not standard, shoppers needed a calculator to compare foods. Many of us just paid attention to the bold slash across the front of the package—"only 5 calories per serving!" We didn't bother to note that a reasonable portion was often far more than the amount the manufacturer called a serving.

Thanks to the Nutrition Labeling and Education Act of 1990, today's food label really helps in making informed decisions. The label's nutrition facts panel can help you budget your calories and determine how much fat, saturated fat, cholesterol and sodium you eat in a day or over the course of several days. Standardized servings level the playing field, and you can trust claims like "low-fat," "high-fiber" and "sodium-free." A list of ingredients is also required on almost all foods, with ingredients listed in descending order by weight. This tool is especially helpful for people with allergies who need to watch out for certain ingredients.

If you've looked carefully at food labels, you have seen the term "% Daily Value." This number tells you how a particular nutrient in a specific food measures up to the amount recommended for your total daily diet. Do you remember the U.S. RDAs for vitamins and minerals? You used to see them on cereal boxes. Basically, % Daily Values (DVs) have replaced those RDAs. You can use % DVs not only to monitor nutrients like fat, which you may want to limit, but also to keep track of nutrients like calcium, which you may want to increase.

There are two key points to remember about DVs. First, they are linked to the serving size listed on the label. If the serving size is 1 cup, but you eat 2 cups, the % DVs double also. Second, Daily Values are based on a 2,000-calorie diet. This particular calorie level is appropriate for moderately active women, teenage girls and sedentary men. If you eat more or fewer than 2,000 calories a day, you have to adjust the DVs accordingly. A nutrition professional can help you do this.

The food label's nutrition panel was a giant step forward in helping us to be smarter consumers and take charge of planning healthy diets. But as soon as the first label encircled the first can, there were comments about what the nutrition panel fails to do. For example, the controversy over trans fatty acids heated up just as the label was approved. Some scientists and nutrition advocates believe that trans fatty acids should be singled out on the label under fat, the same way saturated fat is. But because of limited information about their biological effects, trans fatty acids have not been added to the nutrition facts panel.

If you are concerned about trans fat (found in stick margarine, some fried fast foods and some prepared baked goods), check the ingredient list on the food labels for partially hydrogenated oils. That's where the trans fatty acids mostly are. Since ingredients are listed in descending order by weight, where hydrogenated fat appears on the list gives some indication of how much trans fat there is in the food's overall fat content.

Some of the most nutritious foods don't even have a label. For example, fresh fruits and vegetables and food sold in bulk—like grains, nuts and dried fruits—are exempt from labeling laws. And even though you can now trust a label that says "low-fat," don't be fooled into thinking you're getting "low-calorie" in the bargain. Reduced-fat or fat-free foods—like cookies, for example—are very high in calories (mostly from added sugar).

Nutrition Facts

Serving Size 1 cup (248g)
Servings Per Container 4

Amount Per Serving

Calories 150   Calories from Fat 35

	% Daily Value*
Total Fat 4g	**6%**
Saturated Fat 2.5g	**12%**
Cholesterol 20mg	**7%**
Sodium 170mg	**7%**
Total Carbohydrate 17g	**6%**
Dietary Fiber 0g	**0%**
Sugars 17g	
Protein 13g	

Vitamin A 4%	•	Vitamin C 6%
Calcium 40%	•	Iron 0%

* Percent Daily Values are based on a 2,000 calorie diet. Your daily values may be higher or lower depending on your calorie needs:

		Calories:	2,000	2,500
Total Fat	Less than		65g	80g
Sat Fat	Less than		20g	25g
Cholesterol	Less than		300mg	300mg
Sodium	Less than		2,400mg	2,400mg
Total Carbohydrate			300g	375g
Dietary Fiber			25g	30g

Reading the Nutrition Facts Panel

The food label can help you make informed food choices. Use it to understand how all foods—including your favorites—fit into a healthful diet, one that includes moderate amounts of a variety of foods.

Serving Size. Serving size is based on a typical portion as determined through consumer surveys conducted by the U.S. government. All the other information on the panel about the food relates to this serving size.

Amount per Serving. The numbers next to the nutrients listed in this part of the panel are simply weights, measured in grams (g) or milligrams (mg). They show how much of each nutrient a serving contains.

Vitamins and Minerals. All labels must list the % Daily Value for four key vitamins and minerals: vitamin A, vitamin C, calcium and iron. If other vitamins or minerals have been added or if the product makes a claim about other vitamins or minerals, their % Daily Value also must be listed.

Calories and Calories from Fat. In addition to the total calories contained in a serving of the food, the panel also lists how many of the calories come from fat. These amounts alone aren't enough to see how the food fits in a total diet. The rest of the nutrition panel, including % Daily Value, will help you make a decision.

% Daily Value. For a balanced diet, there are recommended daily amounts you should have of each nutrient. The % Daily Value tells you how much of the recommended amount of a nutrient is in a serving of the food. It's important to note, however, that the % Daily Values for fat, cholesterol, sodium and carbohydrate are based on a sample diet of 2,000 calories a day. If you eat more than this, the food would add a lower % Daily Value to your diet. If you eat less than 2,000 calories, the food would add a higher % Daily Value to your diet. The values presented for protein, iron, calcium and vitamin A are fixed and independent of calories. For example, the recommended amount of vitamin A for a 1,500- and a 4,000-calorie diet is the same.

Recommended Total Daily Amounts. This section is always the same when it appears on labels. It shows the recommended amount, in grams or milligrams, of each nutrient for two different sample diets—one based on 2,000 calories a day, the other on 2,500.

THE SECRET OF THE PYRAMIDS

The Traditional Healthy Mediterranean Diet Pyramid debuted in 1994 with some impressive credentials. It was developed by the Harvard School of Public Health in partnership with the World Health Organization and the Oldways Preservation and Exchange Trust. About a year later, The Traditional Healthy Asian Diet Pyramid premiered, again developed by Harvard and Oldways, this time in cooperation with Cornell University. Both of these pyramids depict traditional diets from cultures where chronic disease rates are low and life expectancies are high.

The Mediterranean and Asian pyramids and the Food Guide Pyramid share some characteristics, but they differ significantly when it comes to others. Grains are the foundation for all three pyramids, with fruits and vegetables in a prominent place on the second tier. The Mediterranean and Asian pyramids, however, separate the plant-based proteins—beans, legumes and nuts—from meat, poultry and fish. From this point upward, the Mediterranean and Asian pyramids differ markedly from the Food Guide Pyramid by giving olive/vegetable oil its own tier and by downplaying dairy foods and red meat.

Proponents of all three pyramids agree that saturated fats should be limited to protect against heart disease. But in the Mediterranean and Asian pyramids, heart-healthy monounsaturated fats, like olive oil and

TRADITIONAL HEALTHY ASIAN DIET PYRAMID

Preliminary Concept
December 1, 1995

This traditional healthy Asian Diet Pyramid reflects Asian dietary traditions historically associated with good health. It is one of a group of food guide pyramids developed through a series of conferences — Public Health Implications of Traditional Diets — that consider diverse dietary traditions around the world. These food guide pyramids, a principal objective of the conferences, are intended to stimulate greater dialogue and interest in cultural models for healthy eating. This Asian Diet Pyramid should be considered preliminary and subject to revision in light of ongoing nutrition research.

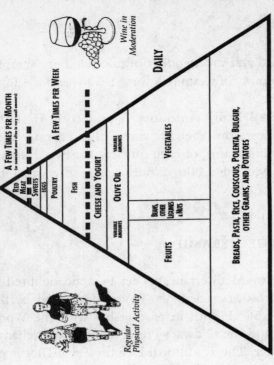

Monthly[1]

Weekly[1]

Optional Daily

Daily

Meat

Sweets

Eggs & Poultry

Fish & Shellfish *or* Dairy[2]

Vegetable Oils

Sake, Wine, Beer, Other Alcoholic Beverages,[3] and Tea

LEGUMES, NUTS, & SEEDS

VEGETABLES

FRUITS

RICE, RICE PRODUCTS, NOODLES, BREADS, MILLET, CORN and other GRAINS[4]

Physical Activity

© 1995 Oldways Preservation & Exchange Trust

(1) Or more often in very small amounts.
(2) Dairy foods are generally not part of the healthy, traditional diets of Asia, with the notable exception of India. In light of current nutrition research, if dairy foods are consumed on a daily basis, they should be used in low to moderate amounts, and preferably low in fat.
(3) Wine, beer and other alcoholic beverages should be consumed in moderation and primarily with meals, and avoided whenever consumption would put an individual or others at risk.
(4) Minimally refined whenever possible.

Preliminary Concept Presented at the
1995 INTERNATIONAL CONFERENCE ON THE DIETS OF THE ASIA
Organized by
Cornell University • Harvard School of Public Health • Oldways Preservation & Exchange Trust

---

THE TRADITIONAL HEALTHY MEDITERRANEAN DIET PYRAMID

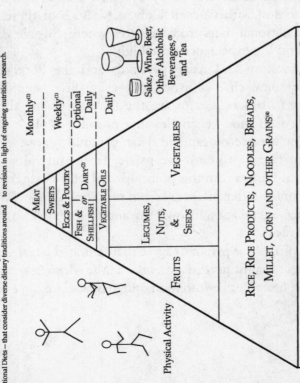

Wine in Moderation

DAILY

A FEW TIMES PER MONTH (or somewhat more often in very small amounts)

A FEW TIMES PER WEEK

RED MEAT

SWEETS

EGGS

POULTRY

FISH

CHEESE AND YOGURT

OLIVE OIL

VARIABLE AMOUNTS

BEANS, OTHER LEGUMES & NUTS

VEGETABLES

FRUITS

BREADS, PASTA, RICE, COUSCOUS, POLENTA, BULGUR, OTHER GRAINS, AND POTATOES

Regular Physical Activity

© Copyright 1994 Oldways Preservation & Exchange Trust.

The Traditional Healthy Mediterranean Diet Pyramid was jointly developed by Oldways Preservation & Exchange Trust, World Health Organization (WHO) European Regional Office, and WHO/FAO Collaboration Center in Nutritional Epidemiology at Harvard School of Public Health. The Mediterranean Diet Pyramid, along with an extensive set of explanatory notes, is available in the form of a large, three-color poster. To receive a copy, please send a check for eight dollars per poster to Oldways Preservation & Exchange Trust, 25 First Street, Cambridge, MA 02141. Telephone 617.621.3000. Fax 617.621.1230.

canola oil, and polyunsaturated fats, like vegetable oil, are positioned as "daily choices." Critics of this approach warn that it's harder to control calories when a diet is high in any kind of fat. And since the Mediterranean and Asian pyramids do not suggest actual servings per day, it's more difficult to use them to plan.

Some experts are also concerned because the Mediterranean and Asian pyramids suggest limiting red meat to only a few times a month and discourage eating dairy products. In my opinion, these two recommendations can be especially troublesome for women because we need the iron, zinc and B vitamins found in meat plus the calcium in dairy products. Mediterranean and Asian pyramid supporters respond that all the nutrients we need are available in a more plant-based diet. In addition, the less protein we eat, the less calcium we need because protein, especially from animal sources, accelerates calcium loss in the urine.

Faced with all three pyramids, what should you do? I agree with my colleagues who caution that the Mediterranean and Asian pyramids promote a diet that is too high in fat for most women. Try to keep fat intake at 30 percent or less of calories, and replace saturated fat with unsaturated vegetable oils such as olive, canola, soybean, corn and safflower oils.

As far as the protein and calcium controversy is concerned: If you are going to eliminate red meat from your diet, be sure you eat enough plant-based proteins, like legumes and beans, to get the nutrients you need. (For example, you need about 50 grams of protein a day, about 60 grams if you're pregnant.) If you are a vegan—that is, if you eat absolutely no animal products, including dairy products or eggs—talk to your physician or a nutrition professional about your need for vitamin B_{12} and vitamin D, two vitamins not found in plant foods. You need vitamin D in order to absorb calcium and vitamin B_{12} to build red blood cells and keep your nervous system healthy.

It is true that if you eat less protein, you may need less calcium. Even without dairy products, it is possible to get enough calcium from foods like almonds, figs, broccoli, kale, and calcium-fortified orange juice, tofu and soy milk. Nevertheless, to be on the safe side, your physician or nutrition professional may advise a calcium supplement. Teenagers, especially girls, often experiment with vegetarianism. Because the adolescent and young adult years are an especially important time for building the bone mass that will prevent osteoporosis, calcium is a primary concern. Make sure the teen girls close to you know how important calcium is to their healthy future.

One more controversial difference between the Mediterranean and Asian pyramids and the Food Guide Pyramid is the presence of alcohol. The Dietary Guidelines for Americans recommend that women limit alcohol to one drink a day—one ounce of spirits, three to four ounces of wine or twelve ounces of beer. Because alcohol is not considered a *necessary* part of a healthy diet, it's not included in the Food Guide Pyramid. Both the Mediterranean and Asian pyramids, however, actually recommend alcohol in moderation as a choice.

This area is one of great controversy. Some studies have shown that alcohol can lower blood's tendency to clot, positively influencing heart health. Other research has linked alcohol to breast cancer, osteoporosis and hypertension. Although moderate drinking may lower the risk for coronary artery disease, heavy drinking can weaken the heart muscle so much that it can no longer pump blood. There also is controversy over what kind of alcohol has positive effects. Some studies point to red wine, others to white wine, still others to both types of wine as well as beer and spirits. Research indicates that alcohol's heart-healthy influence may come from the alcohol itself (ethanol) or, in the case of wine, from compounds found in grapes.

All the publicity about the health benefits of alcohol doesn't mean you should start drinking. But if you drink moderately, there's probably no reason to stop. Do keep in mind, though, that women are especially susceptible to heart and liver damage from alcohol because we don't metabolize it as efficiently as men do.

Drink for drink, more alcohol gets into a woman's bloodstream. In fact, one drink has the same effect on an average-size woman as two have on an average-size man.

And then there are the calories—7 per gram in alcohol, with no real nutritive value. Most drinks contain at least 100 calories; some as many as 200. Even a drink a day in addition to what you already eat could add ten to twenty pounds over the course of a year.

Points to Remember

For high-performance health, rely on your nutrition tool kit:

- ◆ **The Dietary Guidelines—your "owner's manual" for good health**
- ◆ **The Food Guide Pyramid—your blueprint for turning guidelines into food choices**
- ◆ **The food label—your tool for making informed food choices**

MACROS AND MICROS: FEEDING THE ENGINE

The nutrients in the foods you choose fuel your body engine. Think of it this way: The macronutrients—carbohydrate, fat and protein—provide energy; the micronutrients—vitamins and minerals—plus other compounds like phytochemicals keep the engine running smoothly.

We're not going to discuss every nutrient in detail here, but I do want to clear up some confusion about fat and carbohydrates in particular, and highlight some facts that are particularly meaningful to women. For more extensive information, consult *The American Dietetic Association's Complete Food and Nutrition Guide* (Chronimed Publishing, 1996) or call the American Dietetic Association's Nutrition Hot Line at (800) 366-1655.

Fat: Too Much of a Good Thing

In all the hullabaloo about cutting back on fat, we may have lost sight of some of dietary fat's positive attributes. Fat isn't intrinsically "bad." It's a vital nutrient and at nine calories per gram, it's the most concentrated source of calories in the diet. Fat supplies essential fatty acids our bodies can't manufacture. It also maintains healthy skin and hair, regulates levels of cholesterol in the blood and carries the fat-soluble vitamins A, D, E and K.

Many of the chemicals that make food taste good and smell good are carried in fat. The mouth feel or texture of food also is linked to fat. Saturated fats like butter linger on the tongue, providing a satisfying aftertaste, and fat marbled through meat bastes and softens the muscle as it cooks. Fat also makes piecrust tender and flaky and French fries crispy.

We inherited a love of fat from our hunter-gatherer ancestors. When food was scarce, early humans relied on their bodies' stored fat for energy to survive. Naturally, they sought out high-fat foods to build up a good supply of body fat. As time went on, eating high-fat foods became a sign of wealth. Although we don't face the same feast-or-famine challenge as our ancestors, we still crave fat. Because of the abundance of fat in our diet and our increasingly sedentary lifestyle, more dietary fat is stored as body fat, leading to overweight and obesity.

Types of Fat: The fats in food, called triglycerides, contain mixtures of both saturated and unsaturated (polyunsaturated and monounsaturated) fatty acids. In general, when a food contains mostly saturated fat, it's solid at room temperature. When a food contains mostly unsaturated fat, it's usually liquid at room temperature. Most of us know by now that because saturated fat raises blood cholesterol levels, it increases the risk for heart disease. Lately, you may have been hearing that monounsaturated fat is heart healthy. Although there is evidence that monounsaturated fat boosts HDL "good" cholesterol, it's important to remember that all fat, regardless of any other features it may have, has nine calories per gram. Eating too much of *any* fat will contribute to weight gain. So rather than *adding* monounsaturated fat to your diet, use it to *replace* some of the saturated fat you're already eating.

Trans Fatty Acids: You may have been told that for heart health, polyunsaturated fats are a better choice than saturated fats. That advice is still valid, but there is a twist—trans fatty acids. Trans fats are produced when polyunsaturated fat is hydrogenated—that is, when it is chemically altered to become harder and more stable at room temperature. As a result of hydrogenation, polyunsaturated fat becomes more like saturated fatty acid, which is not a healthy choice. Partially hydrogenated polyunsaturated fat is a common ingredient in stick margarine, some fried fast foods and some prepared baked goods like donuts.

Controversy over trans fat abounds. Some researchers maintain that trans fatty acids not only raise LDL "bad" cholesterol but also lower HDL "good" cholesterol and, as a result, contribute to 30,000 of the 500,000 heart disease deaths a year in the USA. Some scientists and consumer advocates believe trans fat should be treated as a separate category on the nutrition panel of the food label. But the consensus among leading health and nutrition organizations is that all the uproar is much ado about relatively little. I agree. If you are following the Food Guide Pyramid, you are probably not eating much trans fatty acid. In fact, trans fatty acids make up only about 2 percent of our calories. Saturated fat, however, which undoubtedly contributes to far more than 30,000 heart disease deaths each year, makes up about 15 percent of our calories.

The best plan is to keep overall fat consumption to 30 percent or less of calories and saturated fat consumption to 10 percent or less of calories. If eating margarine made with partially hydrogenated oil instead of eating butter, which contains saturated fat, helps you do that, fine. If you are especially concerned about trans fatty acids, choose soft or liquid margarines (they contain less hydrogenated oil). Since margarine accounts for only 20 percent of the trans fatty acid in a typical American diet, you can make an even bigger dent in trans fat consumption by limiting processed foods like baked goods. Look for "partially hydrogenated vegetable oil" on the ingredient list and limit these foods.

Omega-3 Fatty Acids: Long before we heard about the dangers of trans fats, we were hearing about the benefits of omega-3s, the polyunsaturated fatty acids found in fatty coldwater fish, such as mackerel, albacore tuna, salmon, sardines, lake trout and, yes, caviar. Omega-3 fatty acids are also found in canola, soy and walnut oils.

Omega-3 fatty acids may help prevent blood clots that can cause heart attack and stroke. They also may help prevent hardening of the arteries. Research suggests that a particular omega-3 fatty acid—docosahexaenoic acid or DHA—may have an effect on brain chemistry, development and functioning. Evidence suggests that DHA helps regulate the "feel good" brain chemical serotonin, and some researchers speculate that DHA may have a protective role in degenerative brain diseases like Alzheimer's that lead to memory loss and dementia. And it seems that DHA may play a role in stress reduction, too, by suppressing the release of damaging stress hormones.

With all this potential good news about fish oil, you might be tempted to take a fish oil capsule, rather than eat the "real thing." But think twice before taking fish oil supplements. They contain a far more potent dose of omega-3 fatty acids than found naturally in food, and we don't know the long-term effects of such high doses. Getting your omega-3s in Mother Nature's package is not only safer but may be more effective because other nutrients and compounds in fish may also have beneficial effects on your health. In addition, substituting fish for fatty meats is an effective way to decrease saturated fat in your diet.

Let me stress again that fat is not bad, but as with any good thing, we can consume too much. We know for a fact that a diet high in saturated fat raises LDL ("bad") cholesterol, thus increasing the risk for heart disease. Health authorities advise keeping your dietary cholesterol intake under 300 grams a day, but it's saturated fat that contributes to high blood cholesterol levels. Since dietary cholesterol is found only in animal products, it tends to go hand in hand with saturated fat. Cutting back on saturated fat will decrease dietary cholesterol.

Cholesterol: Like fat, cholesterol isn't a bad thing. Every cell in your body contains some cholesterol, which is necessary for normal cell function and production of certain hormones. Your liver produces all the cholesterol you need, so it's not an essential nutrient you must get from food. The excess cholesterol circulating in your bloodstream is the problem. Eventually, it builds up on the walls of your arteries and can block blood flow. When the coronary or cerebral arteries are blocked, the result is heart attack or stroke.

The familiar initials LDL and HDL are two types of protein-encased packages called lipoproteins that ferry cholesterol around in your blood. The higher your LDL level, the more cholesterol circulating in your bloodstream. LDL drops cholesterol off where it's needed, but it also deposits excess cholesterol along your artery walls and in other tissues. That's why LDL is characterized as "bad."

The HDL lipoprotein package cleans up the excess cholesterol left by LDL and returns it to the liver. The more HDL you have, the more thorough the cleanup. Consequently, HDL is considered protective or "good." For women, a high triglyceride level may be a better predictor of heart disease than high LDL, and a low HDL level is especially dangerous.

People's response to dietary cholesterol varies. Some are very sensitive to it; others have only a minimal response. But cholesterol levels aren't determined by diet alone. Age, heredity, weight and weight distribution, as well as level of exercise have an impact, too. Smoking, drinking alcohol and taking hormone replacement therapy also can influence cholesterol, especially HDL level. The section on heart disease in chapter 2 explores cholesterol in more detail. What you need to remember is that simply looking at your *total* cholesterol number won't give you the whole story. Ask your doctor for all your numbers—total LDL, HDL and triglycerides—and analyze them in relation to one another. For example, if your total cholesterol is borderline-to-high (200–239), it may be because your HDL level is high. (It should be at least 60.) That's not so bad. But if your total cholesterol is high and HDL is low (less than 35), your situation may be more risky than it appears at first glance.

Fat and Cancer: While the connection between saturated fat and heart disease is well established, the link between fat and cancer—specifically breast and colon cancer—is still inconclusive. A major problem in interpreting these studies is that diets high in fat are usually high in calories, too. It is difficult to determine which is causing the problem. It may be that total calorie intake creates a greater cancer risk than dietary fat. (See the section on breast cancer in chapter 2.)

Fake-Fat Frenzy

In survey after survey, consumers rank taste as their most important consideration in choosing foods. Although many of us are willing to try new products, few of us will buy a product a second time if it doesn't taste good. Food technology continues to develop all sorts of new foods made with ingredient substitutes that remove calories while preserving flavor. Fat replacers are among the most important breakthroughs in food technology.

Fat-reduction ingredients can be carbohydrate-, protein- or fat-based. Real dietary fat contains nine calories a gram, but fat substitutes can contain half that or less. The much-publicized olestra, for example, is a fat-based fat substitute that moves through the digestive tract unabsorbed. Consequently, it is calorie-free.

Proponents claim that fake fats are a positive addition to the food supply because they expand our low-fat and fat-free choices, which is especially helpful for people who need to lose weight. But when you choose foods made with fat substitutes, it is very easy to fall into what I call the "diet soda and hot fudge sundae trap." Be careful not to use low-fat and fat-free foods as an excuse to eat a lot of other high-fat or high-calorie foods.

Carbohydrates: Fueling the Fire

Carbohydrates are the body's main source of energy. In food, carbohydrates can be sugars or starches. But in the body, both types are converted into glucose (blood sugar), the fuel we use to do everything from breathe to run a marathon.

Sugars, like the carbohydrate in fruit or table sugar, are made up of only one or two sugar units. Starches, however, are made up of many sugar units. They're not sweet because their molecules are too big for our taste buds to detect. (If you leave a cracker in your mouth long enough for the digestive enzymes in your saliva to break down the starch into sugar, you'll taste sweetness.)

So if all carbohydrates eventually become glucose in the body, does it make any difference if we get our carbohydrates from sugar or from starch? Yes, in fact, it makes a big difference. Prepared foods containing simple sugars tend to contain a lot of fat and calories and are usually low in vitamins and minerals. In other words, they're not nutrient dense. A number of starchy foods, however, are rich in micronutrients and in the case of beans and legumes, rich in protein as well. Fruits, although they contain the sugar fructose, also are rich in fiber and lots of vitamins. Some foods—whole-grain breads, rice, pasta, beans and vegetables—are good sources of both starch and fiber.

Sugar: Although sugar may not pack the nutrition punch of starch, it has its value. We crave sugar's sweetness the same way we crave fat, and the reasons are likely buried in our evolutionary past.

One theory is that early women (the gatherers of the hunter-gatherer team) used sweetness as an indicator of safety when foraging for food in the wild.

Sugar also plays an important role in kitchen chemistry. It allows yeast doughs to rise, makes cakes light and crumbly, and makes cookies crisp. If you cut back on sugar in fruit jams and jellies, you lose its preservative effect, and mold grows more quickly.

A common myth about sugar is that it causes or aggravates diabetes. We now know, however, that starches and sugars have the same effect on blood sugar. It's the *total* amount of carbohydrate, not the type, that matters in glucose control. The notion that sugar causes hyperactivity in children has been largely abandoned as well.

But sugar does cause weight gain, right? Not really. Like dietary fat, sugar per se does not add extra pounds. Calories do. Although carbohydrates have only four calories per gram, sweet foods are often high in fat, which has nine calories per gram. Low-fat and fat-free products often make up for the lost flavor of fat with more sugar. Consequently, they may contain almost as many calories as their full-fat counterparts. If you crave sugar or the much-loved sugar-fat combination (like chocolate), eat some. If you reasonably satisfy an occasional craving, you'll feel better, have a greater sense of control and avoid potential food binges.

Fiber: Are you wondering if there's something out there that doesn't have calories? There is—fiber. Unfortunately, we don't eat fiber all by itself and probably wouldn't enjoy it much if we did. Fiber is found only in plant food. Because we don't have the enzymes we need to digest it, fiber enters the large intestine intact. Fruit, vegetables, nuts, legumes, brown rice, barley and oats are good sources of soluble fiber. Wheat bran, whole-grain breads and cereals have more insoluble fiber (see sidebar). Because most plant foods contain some of both, it is hard to sort out exactly which type of fiber does what.

Where's the Fiber?		
Food	*Serving Size*	*Grams of Fiber*
High-fiber and bran cereals	1/2 cup	up to 13.5
Baked beans	1/2 cup	8.3
Broccoli, cooked	1 medium stalk	7.4
Spinach, cooked	1/2 cup	5.7
Kidney beans	1/2 cup	4.5
Apple	1 medium	4.5
Banana	1 medium	4.0
Corn	1/2 cup	3.9
Potato	1 medium	3.9
Pear	1 medium	3.8
Lentils	1/2 cup	3.7
Sweet potato	1 medium	3.5
Brown rice, uncooked	1/2 cup	2.8
Peanut butter	2 tablespoons	2.4
Carrots, raw	1 medium	2.3
Peaches	1 medium	2.1
Strawberries	1/2 cup	1.6
Cauliflower, raw	1/2 cup	1.0

Experts aren't sure exactly how much fiber we need. The American Dietetic Association currently recommends twenty-five to thirty grams daily. Scientists know for sure that fiber—especially insoluble fiber—helps prevent constipation. It may also help prevent colon cancer by quickly moving potential carcinogens out of the colon. The colon cancer connection has been hard to prove because there are so many other substances in high-fiber foods that also might have an effect on cancer.

In addition to getting rid of carcinogens, fiber also can cart away valuable minerals like calcium, magnesium, iron and zinc. Most fiber-rich foods, however, have a high-enough mineral content to counterbalance this effect. Fiber supplements do not contain minerals. That is one major reason it is better to get your fiber from food instead of from pills or powders.

Perhaps fiber's biggest claim to fame is its cholesterol-lowering potential. Several years ago, oat bran, which is rich in soluble fiber, was hailed as a great way to lower the risk of heart disease. Subsequent studies challenged oat bran's positive effect on people with *normal* cholesterol levels. Now it appears that oat bran—1 3/4 cups of cooked oatmeal or 1 cup of cooked oat bran daily—can help lower elevated LDL ("bad") cholesterol levels without lowering HDL ("good") cholesterol. Experts caution, however, not to zero in on oats at the expense of other fibers. Remember to strive for balance and variety!

Fiber also helps in weight control. When saturated with water in the stomach, fiber makes us feel full. If you increase your fiber intake gradually, you shouldn't be bothered with gas and bloating. For fiber to be most effective, drink at least eight glasses of water a day. Without enough water, fiber can slow or even block digestion.

Calories Do Count!

Despite a growing reliance on low-fat and fat-free foods, Americans are gaining weight. According to the National Center for Health Statistics, 35 percent of women over age twenty are overweight. Thirty years ago, twenty years ago, even as recently as ten years ago, the number was only 25 percent. What happened? Calories happened.

Although fat intake has gone from 36 percent of calories to 34 percent in the last decade, calorie consumption has gone up by about 230 calories a day. So even though our diet percentages are looking better, we are actually eating more calories and, gram for gram, the same amount of fat. In addition, most people don't get a lot of exercise, so it's not surprising to see those pounds add up.

It may be that the low-fat and fat-free foods that were designed to help us lose or maintain our weight are helping us gain pounds instead—simply because we eat too many of them. The extra carbohydrates we take in from overindulging in these foods just add up to more calories than we can burn off.

VITAMINS AND MINERALS: HIGH-PERFORMANCE BOOSTERS

While macronutrients like fat and carbohydrate fuel the body's engine, micronutrients—vitamins and minerals—keep things running smoothly and efficiently.

Antioxidants: The antioxidant vitamins A, C and E, plus carotenoids and the mineral selenium, have been in the headlines on a fairly regular basis. Antioxidants may help prevent a number of diseases, like cancer and heart disease, and may slow the aging process by neutralizing highly unstable free radical molecules that wreak havoc on the body's cells and membranes. Free radicals are the by-product created by the body's cells as they process oxygen.

You wouldn't suspect it from all the press coverage antioxidants receive and all the supplements on retail shelves, but we don't really know which antioxidants do what, how they do it or what an optimal intake is. It may be that antioxidants work differently, depending on their location in the body and the presence of other nutrients or compounds like phytochemicals (see sidebar on the following page).

Those Fabulous Phytochemicals

Not only are they on the frontier of nutrition research and one of the hottest health topics, phytochemicals also are one of the best arguments for eating a variety of foods. Found in plant-based foods, phytochemicals are non-nutrient compounds that may help protect against heart disease and certain cancers. They also may lower high blood pressure and cholesterol and even fight off viruses. In earlier chapters, I've referred to phytoestrogens, which are plant-based hormones found primarily in soy foods. Phytoestrogens—there are at least fifteen of them—are a type of phytochemical.

There are thousands of phytochemicals. Scientists have already identified about 3,000 with potential health benefits. Eating a wide variety of vegetables, fruits and grains will expose you to a wide range of phytochemicals—even some that scientists have yet to discover. Eventually, we will learn what foods are particularly dense in phytochemicals. But we don't have to understand the function of every phytochemical to know that eating a lot of plant-based foods has tremendous health benefits. Orange juice alone contains fifty-nine known phytochemicals. Garlic and onions have at least fifty.

As you might expect, phytochemically fortified foods are currently being developed and supplements already are on the market. As with vitamins and minerals, it's better (and less expensive) to get phytochemicals from the food in which they naturally occur. If you rely on supplements, you'll be limiting yourself to known phytochemicals only—and to only some of them at that.

Here is a list of some of the most common phytochemicals and the foods in which they are found. These particular phytochemicals are thought to protect against heart disease and/or cancer.

A Few Phytochemicals

Substance	*Sample Food Sources*
Indoles	Cruciferous vegetables, such as broccoli, cabbage, kale
Phytoestrogens	Soybeans, tofu and other legumes
Polyphenols:	
Flavonoids	Citrus fruits, onions, apples, grapes, wine, tea
Isoflavones	Soybeans, other legumes, licorice
Catechins	Tea
Saponins	Garlic, onions, licorice, legumes
Phenolic acids	All plants
Protease inhibitors	Soybeans and all plants
Carotenoids	Orange, red, yellow fruits, many green vegetables
Capsaicin	Chili peppers
Lignans	Flaxseed, berries, whole grains, licorice

Some studies have shown that when LDL cholesterol is exposed to free radicals, it becomes even more damaging to arteries. Antioxidant vitamins may help prevent this damage, lowering the risk for heart disease. Research also suggests that antioxidants may protect against cancer, but these findings are still controversial. In addition, some scientists believe that age-related macular degeneration, a leading cause of blindness in older adults, may be prevented and treated with antioxidant vitamins. And there is evidence to indicate that antioxidants may prevent or delay cataracts as well.

Most of the data that link antioxidants to disease prevention come from large population surveys or from laboratory and animal studies—none of which tell what antioxidants really do in humans. Several major clinical trials now under way are likely to clarify the role antioxidants may play in preventing disease. The findings could have a major impact on our diets and our health.

In the meantime, here's a roundup of what we do know about antioxidants:

- ◆ **Vitamin A/Carotenoids:** We need vitamin A and some carotenoids (which our bodies convert into vitamin A) for proper vision, new cell growth and healthy tissue. Vitamin A also increases resistance to infection. Whereas too much vitamin A can be dangerous, there are no reported adverse effects of very high beta-carotene intakes. The recommended daily vitamin A intake for women is 4,000 international units. Good sources of vitamin A and beta-carotene include dark green leafy vegetables (spinach, kale, broccoli, Brussels sprouts, asparagus), yellow-orange vegetables and fruits (carrots, sweet potatoes, pumpkins, winter squash, cantaloupe, apricots), liver and milk.

- ◆ **Vitamin C:** Vitamin C helps maintain healthy bones, connective tissue and teeth. It also helps increase the absorption of iron and folic acid. The recommended daily intake for vitamin C is 60 milligrams (100 milligrams for smokers). Some scientists believe that the recommended intake should be increased to 200 milligrams daily. When megadoses of vitamin C are consumed, extra vitamin C is simply excreted in the urine. Too much vitamin C isn't toxic but can cause diarrhea. Good sources of vitamin C include citrus fruits and juices, berries, green leafy vegetables, green and red peppers, and tomatoes.

- ◆ **Vitamin E:** A number of researchers believe that vitamin E will eventually prove to be the superstar among all the antioxidants, especially in promoting heart health. Vitamin E helps form blood cells, muscles and healthy lung tissue, and is needed for normal immune system function. The recommended daily intake for vitamin E is 30 international units. It is relatively nontoxic in high doses. Good sources of vitamin

E include whole grains, vegetable oils, egg yolks, liver, wheat germ, nuts, beans, and green leafy vegetables.

◆ **Selenium:** Humans need only small amounts of the mineral selenium, which helps certain enzymes and hormones function. The recommended daily intake for women is fifty-five micrograms. An excess of selenium can be toxic. The selenium content of plant foods varies depending on the selenium content of the soil in which the food is grown. Good sources of selenium include whole-wheat bread, oatmeal, garlic, hazelnuts, tuna, beef, ham, chicken and eggs.

Until research clarifies the role of antioxidants in disease prevention, the smart and safe approach is to make sure foods rich in vitamins A, C, E, beta-carotene and selenium are a part of your daily diet. All sorts of antioxidant supplements are advertised and promoted, but remember that even though some micronutrients are safe in megadoses, others are not. And we really don't know a lot about the long-term effects of high doses of relatively safe vitamins such as vitamin E.

Vitamin D: Antioxidants are important micronutrients, but women also should pay special attention to their changing needs for other vitamins and minerals. For example, older women may have lower levels of vitamin D, which is needed to help the body absorb and use calcium to retain bone. Vitamin D also may help relieve osteoarthritis. The body can manufacture vitamin D from sunlight, but many older people don't spend enough time outdoors, nor do they get enough vitamin D from foods like fortified milk. Some nutrition experts believe that older people should take twice the amount of vitamin D currently recommended—that is, 400 international units versus only 200 international units. As you get older, your physician may want you to take a vitamin D supplement to help protect against both arthritis and osteoporosis, and there's little hazard in doing so.

Supplements: Who Needs Them?
According to the National Research Council, people who can benefit from a supplement include:

◆ Pregnant or nursing women who may need additional iron, folic acid and calcium. Folic acid supplementation is also beneficial from the time a woman starts trying to conceive through the first six weeks of pregnancy. Folic acid has been shown to help prevent neural tube birth defects such as spina bifida.
◆ Women who lose iron because of heavy menstrual flow
◆ Postmenopausal women who do not get enough calcium and vitamin D to help prevent osteoporosis
◆ Strict vegetarians who consume no animal products and whose diets may lack calcium, iron, zinc or vitamin B_{12}
◆ People with chronic illnesses who take medications that reduce appetite or interfere with nutrient absorption

Most nutrition professionals advise getting vitamins and minerals from food where they occur naturally with other nutrients or compounds that can influence absorption and effectiveness. While experts agree that a single multivitamin/mineral supplement taken daily is safe, it is often unnecessary if you are eating a well-balanced diet.

B Vitamins: Your need for B vitamins also changes over time. During your childbearing years, you need enough folic acid to guard against birth defects. Later in life, folic acid—along with vitamins B_6 and B_{12}—may protect against high blood levels of a chemical called homocysteine, which is linked to heart attack and stroke. A deficiency in vitamin B_{12} later in life also can result in anemia and neurological problems like poor balance and impaired memory. Good sources of B vitamins are whole grains, meat, fish, poultry, beans and dark green leafy vegetables.

Minerals: Calcium is important throughout life, but especially during the teenage and young adult years when peak bone mass is forming. Calcium needs increase during pregnancy and breast-feeding; your physician undoubtedly will prescribe a calcium-containing supplement at this time. Calcium becomes extremely important again during the perimenopausal period and after menopause, especially if you don't take hormone replacement therapy to keep estrogen levels up and help protect your bones. Calcium also improves the action of osteoporosis-fighting drugs. (See chapter 2 for a complete discussion of osteoporosis, chapter 3 for more on nutrition and menopause, and chapter 6 for a close-up on calcium.)

As a companion to calcium and vitamin D, the mineral magnesium is important to bone health. Women should get about 280 milligrams of magnesium daily. Good sources are avocados, wheat germ, nonfat yogurt (also a good calcium source) and dark green leafy vegetables. A magnesium supplement usually is unnecessary.

Iron is yet another mineral with special implications for women. From adolescence to menopause women need almost twice as much iron as men. If you have a heavy menstrual flow, your physician may want you to take an iron supplement. Your need for iron will lessen after menopause, dropping from fifteen to ten milligrams per day. Good sources of iron are lean red meat, kidney beans and tofu.

ARE YOU SALT SENSITIVE?

We appreciate salt for its distinct flavor, but it does more than just taste salty. It enhances the flavor of other ingredients and can actually make some foods taste sweeter. Sprinkled on cucumber slices, for example, salt draws out water, which intensifies natural sugars. Salt also affects the way foods look. For example, it acts as a fixative to keep cooked green vegetables from fading and cauliflower from yellowing.

Chemically, salt is composed of 40 percent sodium and 60 percent chloride, both of which are essential to life. So what is all the fuss about? Our average daily consumption of salt is about 10 grams, or a little more than 1 1/2 teaspoons. This adds up to 4,000 milligrams of sodium—or 3,500 *more* than the 500 milligrams our bodies actually need. For some people, that excess can be very dangerous.

We now know that salt triggers high blood pressure in about 10 percent to 20 percent of people, increasing the potential for heart disease, kidney disease and stroke. What we don't know is who is salt sensitive and who isn't. And, to further complicate things, not everyone who has high blood pressure is salt sensitive. Salt also can play a role in osteoporosis. Researchers have found that high sodium intake leads to high levels of calcium in the urine—calcium that should be in the bones instead.

Sodium should be limited to 2,400 milligrams a day, which is about 6 grams or 1 teaspoon of salt. But if there is a history of high blood pressure in your family, or if, by a process of dietary trial and error, your physician determines you are salt sensitive, you may want to limit your sodium even more. Similarly, if you are at risk for osteoporosis you should consider cutting back on salt. Studies indicate that if you don't keep your sodium under the 2,400-milligrams-a-day limit, you may need as much as 1,700 milligrams of calcium a day to make up for urinary calcium loss.

About 80 percent of the sodium in your diet comes not from the saltshaker but from processed and packaged foods and fast foods—yet another reason to read food labels and to add more fresh fruits and vegetables to your daily fare. Sodium can make a big difference in the way foods taste. So while you are "unlearning" your taste for salt, try reduced-sodium products rather than sodium-free ones. And don't touch the saltshaker until you've tasted your food! As you cut back on salt, you'll actually grow to prefer less.

Processed foods that are especially high in sodium include:

- ◆ **Cured meats,** such as ham, bacon, Canadian bacon, corned beef, and luncheon meats (bologna, salami, turkey loaf and smoked beef)
- ◆ **Commercially prepared products,** such as canned, frozen and dried soup, pickles, frozen dinners, and packaged gravies and sauces
- ◆ **Breakfast-type sausages,** Polish, Italian and Mexican sausages, and hot dogs
- ◆ **Fish** that is commercially frozen, prefried, prebreaded or smoked
- ◆ **Fish** that is canned in oil or brine, such as tuna, salmon and sardines
- ◆ **Canned shellfish** such as shrimp, crab, clams, oysters, scallops and lobster

Points to Remember

For healthy eating:

- ◆ Fat and sugar aren't "bad." They are important nutrients— and they make food taste good. Enjoy both in moderation.
- ◆ Extra calories, regardless of their source, add up to extra pounds.
- ◆ Make food your number-one source for vitamins and minerals. Take only the supplements you really need.

CHAPTER 5

Lifestyle "Wear and Tear"

Like any finely tuned, high-performance machine, your body can absorb a lot of wear and tear, but there are consequences. In this chapter, we're going to look at two sources of that wear and tear—stress and chronic dieting—and examine how they can affect your nutritional health.

STRESS: WELCOME TO YOUR WORLD

Can you even imagine a life without stress? Probably not. Most of us can't because we face a variety of pressure situations each day. But stress doesn't have to be all bad. Sometimes it helps us focus on problems and creates the sense of urgency we need to move ahead. But even so-called normal stress takes its toll, both physically and emotionally.

Many of us are overstressed because we have no downtime, no way to escape pressure and to relax. Thanks to cell phones, beepers, fax and E-mail, the old saying "You can run but you can't hide" has become an apt description of our way of life. It seems as if our whole sense of time has changed. A friend recently told me she caught herself standing over her fax machine, frustrated that it wasn't transmitting faster. This kind of reaction isn't surprising when you consider that today's high-tech world is measured in nanoseconds—increments equal to one billionth of a second.

Women's changing role in society has increased the amount of daily stress we face. Twenty-five years ago, more than two-thirds of women with young children did not have paying jobs. Today, almost two-thirds of them do. In more than 60 percent of American families, both parents work outside the house. And the majority of working mothers are back in the labor force before their babies are a year old.

But women are not relinquishing their responsibilities at home. Between her job, child care and housework, the typical working mother labors seventy-six to eighty-nine hours a week. About a quarter of working women also are caring for at least one disabled elderly family member, and some women have left paying jobs to care for an aging relative. Studies show that more than half of these caregivers experience significant degrees of stress. And experts say that as the population ages, elder care will become a normal life experience for many more women.

It's not surprising, then, that in a U.S. Labor Department survey, working women ranked stress as their number-one problem. Identified by almost 60 percent of respondents, stress cuts across income and occupational groups and is especially acute among women in their forties who have managerial jobs (74 percent) and for single mothers (67 percent). Today, there are close to fifty-nine million working women—almost half of the entire workforce. The U.S. Labor Department predicts that 99 percent of American women will work for pay at some point in their lives. That's a lot of stress!

The Effects of Stress

What exactly is stress? Basically, it's your body's response to a particular physical demand or life experience. When your body recognizes a stressor, it has a "flight-or-fight" reaction during which a number of things happen. Your heart rate speeds up and your brain becomes more alert. Digestion slows and your liver begins to make glucose for energy. Your blood clots more easily and the stress hormone cortisol is released to slow down inflammation of wounds.

This fight-or-flight reaction to stress gave our early ancestors the means to escape from danger. Even though we don't face the same dangers, we still have this reflex. In times of danger it's an asset. But when your body has a recurring stress reaction to the accumulated hassles of everyday living, it's bad for your health. For example, because stress causes your blood to clot more easily, you are at greater risk for a heart attack. And an excess of the stress hormone cortisol circulating in your body can boost your blood pressure, leading to hypertension.

We know that extreme physical stress—like burns, severe injury, surgery, high fever and even rigorous exercise—increases the body's metabolic rate. If you don't get enough calories, protein and other nutrients when you experience this kind of stress, you're likely to become malnourished, which leads to a slower recovery from injury or illness. (Surprisingly, this kind of malnutrition happens to quite a few hospitalized patients, and doctors are becoming more aware of the need for early nutrition therapy to prevent it.) Scientists believe that ongoing stress resulting from emotional or psychological pressure—such as juggling too many demands at work and at home—also may put us at risk for malnutrition and lower our resistance to infection.

You probably have heard about so-called miracle cures for stress. For example, licorice root, Siberian ginseng and wild yam extract supposedly lessen the negative effects of too much cortisol. Although we don't have all the answers about the effect of diet on stress, we do know that the human body is far too complex for any magical nutrient to cure stress. But being well nourished overall can strengthen your body, enabling you to handle stress better and, perhaps, helping to prevent stress-related illness.

His and Hers Brains

That men and women react to stress differently is just one of the fascinating gender differences scientists are exploring. For example, thanks to powerful new brain-imaging techniques, scientists have observed that even though women's brains are smaller than men's (because women's bodies are typically smaller than men's), they apparently have more neurons. All these neurons are in areas of the brain devoted to understanding language and recognizing tone of voice.

Part of the bridge between the left and right sides of the brain is also larger in women than in men. This difference may explain why women use both sides of their brain when processing language, much more so than men do. It is this crosstalk between brain hemispheres that may account for women's "intuition" and their ability to read emotions in other people.

Women's Unique Reactions to Stress

Recent studies show that women's reactions to some types of stress may differ from men's. For example, in one study of boys and girls with anxiety, girls had higher levels of the potentially damaging stress hormone cortisol. Researchers also have found that in stressful situations like marital disagreements, women react more quickly and with a more intense fight-or-flight reflex than do their husbands.

Stress hormones also may be connected to weight distribution in women. Studies show that apple-shaped women—women with more central body fat—secrete more stress hormones than pear-shaped women, whose weight is concentrated in the hips and thighs. Central body fat is known to be a risk factor for heart disease (see chapter 2). In addition, because stress increases blood pressure and heart rate, it is especially harmful to postmenopausal women who no longer are benefiting from the heart-protective effects of estrogen.

Another serious result of chronic stress is depression. People who are depressed sometimes display the same fight-or-flight hormone levels as people under continuous stress. In women, depression rates start to climb at puberty and peak during the childbearing years. This pattern suggests that fluctuating estrogen levels also play a role in depression—perhaps triggering or exacerbating symptoms in women who have a genetic predisposition to the disease. Twice as many women as men are diagnosed with depression. (The rate of substance abuse among men, however, is five times greater than women's and may contribute to keeping their diagnosed rate of depression lower.)

Food Cravings and Stress

When the stress hormone cortisol is released, it triggers a complex interaction of brain chemicals. As a result, levels of the "feel-good" brain chemical serotonin drop, producing a craving for carbohydrates. (You may experience similar food cravings right before your period starts. The physical reason is the same—low serotonin levels in the brain—but rather than stress hormones causing the dip, it's lowered estrogen levels.)

Often, we satisfy these cravings with sweet, high-calorie foods—like chocolate. Researchers speculate that we crave these foods because fat and sugar stimulate the brain to release morphinelike endorphins—the same brain chemical that makes you feel calm after vigorous exercise. Plus sugar triggers a pleasurable serotonin boost. Chocolate also contains several stimulants as well as other druglike compounds that can effect mood. Some scientists, however, are skeptical of chocolate's much ballyhooed mood-altering powers and remind us that cheddar cheese, salami and pickled herring contain even more of these druglike "magic ingredients." But few of us are dying for a slice of salami.

There's nothing wrong with satisfying a food craving with a creamy sweet like chocolate. In fact, if you deny your cravings, you're likely to add to your stress and end up bingeing later. The key is moderation. It doesn't take a whole bag of peanut M & M's to kill the craving. Have a small piece of chocolate rather than an entire chocolate bar. And there is some potential good news about chocolate: Even though it is high in saturated fat, the particular type of saturated fat (stearic acid) it contains does not raise cholesterol levels.

What to Do About Stress and Diet

The degree to which mood can be altered with food is a matter of heated debate among researchers and is likely to be the subject of scientific inquiry for years to come. In the meantime, what nutritional steps can you take now to lessen the effects of stress on your body and keep yourself on an even keel?

If you often crave carbohydrates, try eating small meals (don't forget breakfast!) and snacks throughout the day that include carbohydrates such as whole-grain breads and starchy vegetables. You'll not only keep your cravings in check, you'll also avoid the extra fat and calories that come from eating too much. And if you lose your appetite when you're under stress, eating a series of small meals will be easier than trying to consume several big ones. Remember that stress slows digestion, but the fiber in grains, fruit and vegetables will help keep your digestive system functioning normally. Be sure to drink a lot of water, too.

Remember, you don't have to give up your favorite sweets. Including a couple of sweet snacks in your day will help you avoid bingeing later. If you're a chocolate lover, have some for dessert after a meal when you're less likely to overdo it. During times of stress, you also might want to boost your exercise level. Exercise can stimulate the release of calming endorphins—without those extra calories from chocolate.

We know that vitamin C, vitamin E and the B vitamins can be depleted by stress, but remember one important fact: You can meet virtually all your nutrient needs with a healthy diet. (Exceptions include prenatal vitamin supplements for pregnant women and calcium supplements for postmenopausal women.) Most nutrition professionals believe you don't need to take specially formulated supplements that contain many times over the recommended amount of vitamins and minerals. These products are not advertised as aggressively as they were in the past, but they are still available. Although most won't hurt you, if you neglect your diet in favor of a randomly formulated supplement, you may not get all the nutrients you need.

Points to Remember

To relieve stress and help prevent stress-related disease:

- ◆ **Keep your body well nourished overall. Don't rely on single nutrients to fight stress.**
- ◆ **Eat small meals rich in whole grains and starchy vegetables throughout the day.**
- ◆ **Boost your exercise level.**

DIETING: A LOSING PROPOSITION

In surveys taken twenty-five years ago, only about a quarter of American women said they were unhappy with their appearance. Today, that number has doubled. In a 1996 poll conducted by *People* magazine, women were three times as likely as men to have negative thoughts about their bodies. Weight is the primary concern for many.

Unfortunately, a number of Americans link being overweight to some kind of moral measurement of a person's worth, which easily leads to prejudice and discrimination. It hasn't always been this way. Negative attitudes toward overweight people are largely a twentieth-century phenomenon.

Changing Attitudes

Prior to 1900, in times when food was scarce, being overweight was a sign of prosperity. In the 1800s, many medical experts believed that some extra weight gave people a reserve to fall back on in case of disease or injury.

Attitudes began to change when the vegetarian Sylvester Graham (of cracker fame) became a popular health lecturer. When he equated gluttony—to him, the greatest evil—with obesity, the moral die was cast. There was a brief backlash in the Victorian era when eating a lot and weighing a lot were not only acceptable, they were admired.

By the early 1900s, however, cartoons and jokes about overweight people were common. Fat people were considered ugly. The growing social pressure to be thin created a market for all sorts of gimmicks including appetite suppressants, bath salts and mechanical devices.

Insurance data on weight gain and mortality published in 1912 linked obesity to health for the first time. In 1918, Los Angeles physician and newspaper columnist Lulu Hunt Peters wrote *Diet and Health with a Key to the Calories*. It was America's introduction to calories and how to count them and the first of the diet-book bestsellers. Peters instructed her readers (mostly women) to use the word *calorie* frequently, as in "100 calories of bread" rather than "1 slice of bread." Her approach to dieting actually was quite modern. She advised 1,200 calories per day: 10 percent to 25 percent protein, 25 percent to 30 percent fat, and 60 percent to 65 percent carbohydrate.

In the 1920s and 1930s, the idea that obesity might be purely hereditary temporarily quieted moral judgments about being overweight. When the genetic link failed to provide all the answers, being fat was once again deemed bad and ugly. The fashionable flapper look of the 1920s came at the cost of painful chest-binding, overexercise and starvation diets. The eating disorders anorexia and bulimia first emerged as major health issues at this time.

By the 20s and 30s, movies had become an entertainment staple and film stars were growing in popularity. Everybody wanted to look like a movie star—thin. The Hollywood 18-Day diet became the rage. It was a 585-calorie-a-day regimen of grapefruit, oranges, melba toast, green vegetables and hard-boiled eggs. Also popular at the time was the first of the liquid diets: six bananas blended with three cups of milk, served in small portions throughout the day.

In the 1940s, the emphasis shifted toward measuring body fat rather than counting calories. Psychology was an emerging medical specialty, and being overweight was treated as a problem related to fear, depression, insecurity, sexual repression and oral fixation. Self-help groups became popular at this time. Fat people often were regarded as lacking in willpower and even mentally handicapped.

The diet-food industry took off like crazy in the 1950s. Sales of 900-calorie-per-day liquid diets skyrocketed. Gaylord Hauser's 1950 bestseller *Live Younger, Live Longer* advocated a pound-a-day weight-loss program using a high-protein, low-carbohydrate diet. By 1955, thousands of women were visiting Slenderella Salons, vibrating their fat away on machines—or so they thought—for $2 a session. Despite all this activity, polls taken during the 50s show that people didn't think they were doing much to lose weight. Dieting had become such a routine part of life, people didn't even realize they were doing it.

In the 1950s, television began to exert a profound influence on attitudes about weight and body image. With the introduction of mass media, people could experience life beyond their own communities, and the country began to develop a national standard of what was "normal." In terms of body size, normal meant thin. And thin became thinner in the 1960s and 1970s. Thanks to models like the aptly named Twiggy, the diet industry continued to flourish.

In 1963, Weight Watchers was founded by a New Jersey housewife and promoted sound weight-management techniques. Women's magazines ran more and more articles on dieting. The first big diet book of the 60s was Dr. Herman Taller's *Calories Don't*

Count. Taller maintained that polyunsaturated fat helped melt away body fat. After it was discovered that Taller owned an interest in the mail-order company he recommended as a source for vegetable-oil capsules, he was convicted on twelve counts of mail fraud.

Dr. Irwin Stillman followed Taller in 1967 with *The Doctor's Quick Weight Loss Diet* and Robert Atkins published *Dr. Atkins' Diet Revolution* in 1972. Both Stillman's and Atkins' books recommended diets similar to Taller's, but with slightly lower fat levels. In 1978, the high-protein diet returned with Dr. Herman Tarnower's *The Complete Scarsdale Medical Diet.* By the end of the 1970s, any dieter worth her protein knew the drill: The fewer the carbohydrates the better the fat burn, and never mind the kidney damage that might result.

When Nathan Pritikin established the first of his centers and introduced the Pritikin Diet in the mid 1970s, the pendulum swung back to a low-fat, low-protein regimen with 80 percent of calories coming from carbohydrates. Pritikin's initial audience was composed primarily of executive men fearful of heart disease. Eventually, however, men and women flocked to the Pritikin Diet.

By 1980, a weight-loss frenzy had taken hold of the country. By mid-decade, more than a third of all adults were dieting—trying just about anything from the *Beverly Hills Diet* (nothing but fruit before noon) to the Rice Diet (fruit and rice for weeks). As we entered the 90s, it was no longer enough to be thin; muscle tone mattered, too.

By 1994, everyone from Richard Simmons to Susan Powter to Dean Ornish to Jane Fonda was singing the same low-fat tune, and virtually every dieter—every eater, really—understood that fat has more calories than either carbohydrate or protein. Consequently, people were gobbling up reduced-fat and fat-free foods faster than manufacturers could fill supermarket shelves. Fat consumption went down, but calorie consumption went up.

Today, Dr. Atkins is back with his *New Diet Revolution,* Barry Sears is on the best-seller list with *The Zone* and Adelle Puhn is pushing *The 5 Day Miracle Diet*. All three books are promoting the high-protein diet popular in the 1970s. But you still won't lose weight for good by following these plans. They will result in a dramatic loss of body water at first, which is often mistaken for weight loss. Their long-term effect on the kidneys can be dangerous, especially for older people and for people with undiagnosed diabetes.

The Realities of Dieting

Today's average female store mannequin is a size six and stands five feet ten inches tall. Her measurements are 34-24-34. Here's a reality check: Nearly 50 percent of American women wear a size 14 or larger. Almost a third wear a size sixteen or larger. The average U.S. female is five feet four inches tall and weighs 142 pounds. She has thirty-seven-inch hips. But flying in the face of this reality is relentless pressure to be thin. While there's certainly nothing wrong with wanting to look good, we must work hard to keep a *healthy* perspective on this issue.

When you live a life of chronic dieting rather than healthy eating, you subject your body to a lot of wear and tear. Many people lose weight repeatedly, only to gain it all back—repeatedly. This process is known as weight cycling or yo-yo dieting. Whether or not weight cycling is physiologically harmful is a matter of debate among medical experts. For years, weight cycling was considered harmful because it supposedly permanently decreased the rate at which the body burns calories, made it much harder to lose weight with each successive effort, created more fat and less muscle tissue, instilled a desire for fatty foods, and increased risk for heart disease and diabetes. Some experts maintained that in terms of health risk, remaining overweight was preferable to yo-yo dieting.

But in 1995, after a government panel of experts reviewed thirty years of human research on weight cycling, the verdict changed: Evidence supporting the adverse health effects of yo-yo dieting was weak at best. People who are seriously overweight are now advised

In the Eye of the Beholder

What's considered the body beautiful in a given era is the result of a fairly complex interplay of cultural and societal trends. We happen to live in a time when looking like Cindy Crawford at five feet nine inches, 120 pounds and 34-24-34 is preferred over Twiggy's 1960s five-foot-six-inch body at 92 pounds and 31-22-32.

When Miss Universe 1996 gained some weight, there was talk of taking away her crown. After all, didn't she look a little chubby in that swimsuit? Never mind that at her winning weight and height—five feet seven inches and 112 pounds—Miss Universe met a medical standard for anorexia. Even at 130 pounds, she still weighed less than what is recommended for her height. Just who is making all these dumb rules about size, shape and beauty? How did we get from a voluptuous size-12 Marilyn Monroe ideal in the 1950s to today's size-6 supermodel?

Anthropologists say that, traditionally, men have been judged by what they do and women by how they look—especially when a woman's looks say something about how successful her male companion is. A plump wife, for example, once symbolized her husband's wealth and power, and her curvy figure symbolized her job—childbearing. During periods of dramatic social change for women—for example, in the 1920s when women got the vote and in the 1960s when birth control pills hit the market—the ideal female shape changed to a slimmer profile, one that deemphasized symbols of childbearing like breasts and wide hips. In the 1990s, the emphasis is still on the lean look, but breasts and hips are okay again, as long as they are part of a tall, sculpted athletic shape—in other words, lean and *strong*.

to try to lose weight—even just five or ten pounds and even if they must "yo-yo" a few times to do it.

But there is one negative effect of weight cycling that virtually all experts agree upon: the adverse psychological impact. People who gain and lose weight over and over again may become discouraged. Depression and an erosion of self-esteem are not unusual. But this could be a chicken-and-egg situation: Which comes first—the emotional stress or the weight cycling?

Chronic dieting can be especially hard on a woman's psyche when she's also in charge of planning, shopping for and preparing family meals—especially holiday celebrations that often focus on food as a symbol of togetherness. This "push-me/pull-me" tension creates anxiety and anger that easily leads to depression.

Unfortunately, we still don't have the final word on the effects of yo-yo dieting. For example, in the long run, we don't really know what happens to obese people when they become thin by dieting. Do they enjoy the same health benefits as naturally thin people? It's difficult to find an adequate sample to study when so many formerly obese people gain back the lost weight. We do know, however, that obesity definitely increases risk for many deadly diseases and that starvation diets place dangerous stress on the body. For now, I believe the best advice is to try to avoid the yo-yo syndrome by losing excess weight slowly—about one-half to one pound a week. Become a healthy eater, not a dieter.

Reaching and maintaining a healthy weight has a lot to do with counting calories, and balance is the key. Simply put, take in too many calories and you gain weight; take in too *few* and you may also *gain* weight. That is because when you drastically reduce your calorie intake, your body thinks it's starving and immediately slows down the rate at which you burn calories for fuel. This starvation response is an evolutionary adaptation that helped early humans survive during times of famine. The key to weight *maintenance* is to take in just enough calories to fuel your basic metabolic needs. If you do, your body burns what it needs at a normal rate and there are few calories left over to store as fat. The key to weight *loss* is to reduce calories modestly through diet and exercise to achieve a slow, steady weight loss.

Some scientists believe your body has a certain set point that controls your weight (see chapter 2). When you lose weight, your body compensates by lowering your metabolism so that it's easier for you to gain the weight back. Conversely, when you gain weight, your body speeds up your metabolism in order to burn off fat so you get back to your set point. Researchers speculate that slow weight loss combined with ongoing exercise to build calorie-burning muscle may be the only way to adjust your set point, which may be determined during infancy or even genetically.

Eating Disorders

The desire to achieve a cultural ideal of thinness drives many women to diet severely. For some especially vulnerable women, this behavior leads to eating disorders like anorexia, bulimia, binge eating and chronic dieting. In developing countries where dieting is becoming a fad, doctors are encountering more and more formerly infrequently seen eating disorders.

Adolescent girls—even those as young as age ten or eleven—are especially vulnerable to the body-image pressure our society places on females (see chapter 3). Studies show that half of girls dislike their bodies by age thirteen, and eight out of ten are unhappy with their bodies by age eighteen. Of the estimated eight million people in the United States who suffer from eating disorders, the vast majority began their struggle before age twenty. Ironically, it is just at the time a young girl is most vulnerable to negative messages about her appearance that her body begins to change with the added fat of puberty. Young boys' bodies also change at puberty, but they're not interested in staying slim as much as becoming strong and muscular.

The most common eating disorder is the binge-and-purge disease called bulimia. A bulimic might consume as many as 20,000 calories in a binge lasting eight hours, then use a laxative or diuretic, induce gagging, or take a commonly available over-the-counter medication to induce vomiting. This bingeing and purging leads to a temporary reduction in anxiety and stress. Between binges, the bulimic may fast or exercise excessively. A more recently recognized eating disorder is binge eating that is not followed by a purge. These binge eaters often become obese.

Anorexia is much rarer than bulimia and can be fatal. People with anorexia starve themselves to death while believing they are overweight. Anorexics also may binge and purge and often exercise excessively.

Eating disorders are much more common in women than in men. One simple reason is that women diet more than men. Men are less dependent on their body shape as a definition of masculinity. But most women struggle with body image throughout their lives to a certain degree. A woman with a negative body image is far more likely to perceive her entire self as negative.

You Can't Fool Mother Nature

As body shapes fall in and out of fashion, Mother Nature safeguards one evolutionary mandate: propagation of the species. Healthy, fertile women usually have a waist-hip ratio (WHR) of .6 to .8, even though their weight may vary. In other words, the preferred shape for successful childbearing is one in which waist measurement is between 60 percent and 80 percent of hip size (waist ÷ hip = WHR). No matter how size goes in and out of fashion, attractive *shape* remains fairly constant. From a purely evolutionary perspective, it's no coincidence that men tend to favor this particular female body proportion. Researchers have documented that even as Miss America winners got leaner from 1923 to 1990, their waist-hip ratios stayed between .68 and .78. Even Twiggy had a .68 WHR. Marilyn's was .63 and Cindy's is .7. You just can't fool Mother Nature.

Many women go through life with what are called subclinical eating disorders. These women don't exactly fit all the diagnostic criteria for an eating disorder, but their eating patterns and preoccupation with food are abnormal enough to disrupt their lives and threaten their health. For example, teenage girls who continually restrict their calorie intake may not get enough calcium to build the bone mass they need to prevent osteoporosis in later life.

Some women have only one brief episode of disordered eating— often tied to a traumatic life experience, for example. Others suffer from chronic eating disorders that come and go throughout their lives. Chronic dieting is not the only cause behind eating disorders. Inability to cope with a life situation like pressure at school or work, or the death of a loved one can trigger disordered eating. Some studies suggest there may be a significant genetic link. Eating disorders also may be connected to depression and to a low level of the brain chemical serotonin (see the discussion of stress earlier in this chapter). Just as the causes of eating disorders are complex, so are the treatments, which usually include some combination of individual psychotherapy, group therapy, family counseling, antidepressant drugs, medical nutrition therapy and, perhaps, hospitalization for life-threatening complications.

If you think you might have an eating disorder, ask yourself the following questions. If you answer yes more often than no, seek help right away.

- Do you restrict your calories to fewer than 500 a day or regularly skip two or more meals a day?
- Do you horde food or hide it?
- Do you eat large amounts of food in a short time and feel out of control as you do?
- Do you eat large amounts of food when you aren't hungry?
- Do you feel guilty, depressed or disgusted with yourself after overeating?

- Do you stay at home or avoid people so you can maintain your eating or exercise schedule?
- Do you think food controls your life?
- Do you have an intense fear of gaining weight?

What to Do About Dieting

We will cover more about healthy approaches to weight management and exercise in the next chapter, but for now remember that we have to accept certain social realities, but we don't have to embrace them. For example, society's emphasis on body image isn't going to disappear. What's considered the ideal body may change slightly over time (see sidebar In the Eye of the Beholder, page 149), but it probably will remain unattainable for most women. What we need to strive for is an understanding that social and cultural dynamics do not have to dictate how we feel about ourselves. Getting this message through to young girls and teenagers is especially important.

The multibillion-dollar dieting industry isn't going to disappear, either. There will always be another miracle diet. Most will be recycled or retooled versions of some diet from the past that emphasizes one or two nutrients or a particular food at the expense of balance. As soon as one fad wanes, another will rise up to fill the void, the bookshelves and someone's bank account. If you try these diets, you'll probably lose some weight at first, not because of any magic combination of nutrients, but because you'll lose body water and most likely will be reducing your calorie intake. But in the long run, you can harm your body and your emotional well-being by following a very low-calorie diet or one that stresses a single nutrient or food over others.

When we refer to healthy eating, we're not talking about how thin we are or what diet we're on. We're talking about how what we eat affects our risk factors for various diseases. So the numbers we're really interested in aren't pounds and inches; they are percent of body fat, waist-hip ratio, cholesterol and triglyceride levels, and bone density.

When we take a healthy approach to eating, we also assume responsibility for our own well-being. If you get too hung up on the "rules" of a diet, you may become so out of touch with your body that you no longer know what *real* hunger feels like. Relying on diet books and weight-loss plans to make decisions about what you eat cuts you off from the real world of food. Foods aren't good or bad. They're just food. And eating isn't a moral choice. What you eat doesn't make *you* good or bad.

Remember that a healthy approach to eating is about more than food. It takes into account the whole person—the fact that you are a woman, your age, your level of stress, your genes, your food preferences, your medical history, etc. No simple formula approach to eating could possibly accommodate all these variables. It is precisely because you are a work in progress that your nutrition needs and health change over time.

Points to Remember

To avoid the consequences of chronic dieting:

- ◆ **Make your goal healthy eating rather than being thin.**
- ◆ **Remember that fad diets are rarely healthy diets.**
- ◆ **Know the signs of a potential eating disorder.**
- ◆ **Remember that healthy eating is about more than food; it's about your unique needs, preferences and lifestyle.**

CHAPTER 6

What You Can Do

*N*o more talking about it. Now you are going to *do* it. Knowing the diseases you as a woman are particularly vulnerable to, given the nutrition tools available to you and knowing the built-in stresses of everyday living—here's what I suggest you do:

◆ Maintain a healthy weight.
◆ Enjoy physical activity.
◆ Rebalance your diet. Enjoy more fruit, vegetables and grains and less fat.
◆ Get enough calcium.

As you learn more about these strategies in the pages that follow, you will see that they are closely interwoven. You can pick any one strategy as your starting point and the others will naturally follow.

These strategies work because they are based on the three core principles I outlined in the introduction: balance, variety and moderation. So-called healthy eating plans without this foundation eventually collapse. The novelty wears off, you don't achieve your goal and you are left frustrated and unhappy.

Although balance, variety and moderation are key components of this approach, there's one more critical ingredient: How *ready* are you to make some long-term changes?

Psychologists who study "readiness" say we usually go through a series of stages when we make a lifestyle change. And if we try to make a change before we're ready, failure is likely. How ready are you to change to a healthier way of eating?

THE STAGES OF CHANGE

Adapted from *Changing for Good,* James O. Prochaska, Ph.D., John C. Norcross, Ph.D., and Carlo C. DiClemente, Ph.D., copyright © 1994 by James O. Prochaska, Ph.D., John C. Norcross, Ph.D., and Carlo C. DiClemente, Ph.D. (by permission of William Morrow and Company, Inc.)

- ◆ **Precontemplation:** You haven't given much thought to making a change. You may think you don't need to or that your situation is hopeless. If you embark on any kind of change in this frame of mind, you are likely to fail. Chances are you're doing it not for yourself but to please someone else. This is a good time to seek more information.

- ◆ **Contemplation:** You probably know you'd be healthier if you changed your eating and exercise habits. But you are not sure it's worth the effort. It's easy to get stuck in this stage. To get moving, write down everything you eat for a few days and keep track of your physical activity, too. Consider meeting with a nutrition professional to help you analyze how healthy your habits are—or aren't.

- ◆ **Preparation:** You're thinking more about the future than the past, more about what's possible rather than impossible. You know you need to change, and perhaps you've started to make a few adjustments in your diet. Now is a good time to consider how your lifestyle might interfere with changes you want to make. For example, how will you fit exercise into your schedule? What will you do when you travel or eat out?

◆ **Action:** You're not just *acting* like a woman who follows a healthy diet and gets enough physical activity. You *are* that woman. Now, make sure you get the support you need from your family and friends. Enjoy the feeling of empowerment that comes with taking charge of your nutritional health. Reward yourself!

◆ **Maintenance:** You know what it takes to eat a healthy diet and to get enough exercise every day. Your old habits are gone. But maintenance is a lifelong process, and many people don't succeed in making drastic life changes on their first try. If you slip back into old eating and exercise habits, try to learn from the experience and start again—even if you have to go all the way back to the precontemplation stage.

As you move through the stages of change toward and beyond the action steps I've outlined here, you will continue to be bombarded with information on new research. I hope I have given you some context into which you can place and assess all those miracle cures and magic nutrients. Keep in mind that if it sounds too good to be true, it probably is.

In addition to integrating the action steps that follow into your life, it's important to safeguard your well-being by following a regular schedule of health screenings. Remember that your risk for various diseases changes over time. Regular screenings are a primary form of prevention. (see Your Timetable for Tests: Age Eighteen and Up, pages 161–162).

READING IS BELIEVING?

Just when you thought you had everything under control, they change the rules. Maybe caffeine's not so bad. Maybe margarine's not so good. Who knows!

The media often report on studies published in medical journals as the "final word." No wonder we're confused six months later when the final word changes. Most scientists, however, look at published research as a work in progress. Before a finding becomes a fact it has to be supported again and again, not only in population (also called "epidemiologic") studies and animal studies, but also in properly designed human clinical trials.

When you are evaluating the latest report on a health or nutrition issue, keep these tips in mind.

- ◆ **Consider the source.** The most reliable studies come from major universities, health institutes or health-related associations, and findings are published in peer-reviewed journals like *The Journal of the American Medical Association* or *The New England Journal of Medicine*. In the media, stories reported by medical writers for major publications or news organizations are generally more reliable than those in tabloid newspapers and television. Also consider who funded the research, especially when results support the benefit of a certain food or drug.

- ◆ **Consider the study subjects.** Animal studies are an important part of the total research process, but results from studies on rats don't always apply to humans. In addition, research done exclusively on men or women does not necessarily apply to the other gender. The number of subjects in a study is important, too. Very small studies can yield provocative results but rarely prove anything. Clinical trials typically involve hundreds to thousands of subjects, and population studies involve tens of thousands. How long the study ran is also important, because it may take years to reach a definite conclusion on some issues.

- ◆ **Consider other studies on the same topic.** Rarely can a single study stand on its own. A study that is the first of its kind is less credible than one that supports other research on the same subject. If you've never heard anything about the study topic before, be skeptical.

- **Consider the whole report.** Learn to look behind the headlines. The media love controversy and often put a spin on reports with attention-grabbing headlines. Toward the end of an article or television report, you'll often find the less sensational but broader perspective.
- **Consider your risk before changing your behavior.** Study results don't apply equally to all people; they vary with age, weight, gender, race and other individual characteristics. And when a disease is rare to begin with, increased risk may not mean that much to you. Don't be fooled by *association* between a behavior and a health outcome versus a *cause-and-effect relationship*. Most studies reveal an association. Risks and benefits must be considered together. For example, even if a drug increases some risks, it may reduce other more important ones.
- **Consider what we do know for sure.** It makes more sense to stop smoking, maintain a healthy weight and exercise than it does to avoid a specific food or load up on a particular nutrient.

A final word on information overload and the Internet: Exploring the Internet, you're likely to find hundreds, even thousands, of documents related to any given disease or nutrient. This kind of access to information is good in that it helps us take charge of our own health and well-being, but it also can be dangerous. The Internet is largely unregulated. Anyone can set up a Web site. Use the points I outlined above to help you tell a reliable Web site from a dangerous one. Be particularly wary of sites that promote a specific product, especially if "miracle" claims are made.

Your Timetable for Tests: Age Eighteen and Up

Test	*Time*
Complete physical	• Every 3–5 years
Blood pressure (hypertension)	• As often as you see your physician or at least every other year
	• As required for those on blood pressure medication
Clinical breast examination	• Until age forty, every other year; after age forty, annually
	• Should not replace monthly self-exam
Mammogram	• Every other year during forties, or annually if at high risk
	• Annually after age fifty
Pap smear (cervical cancer)	• Yearly from age eighteen to twenty
	• Every other year after age twenty, or annually if at high risk
	• After standard hysterectomy, every three years (some cervical tissue can remain)
	• Screen for sexually transmitted diseases at the same time, if necessary/appropriate
Pelvic exam	• Until age forty, every other year; after age forty, annually
Cholesterol test (total, LDL, HDL, triglycerides)	• Every five years; more often if monitoring high LDL or triglycerides or low HDL
Colorectal screen (colon cancer)	• Fecal occult blood test: from age forty to fifty, every other year; after 50, annually
	• Digital rectal exam: after age forty, annually

	• Sigmoidoscopy: after age fifty, every other year; yearly if at high risk
Bone density	• For those at risk for osteoporosis, during forties
	• Establish baseline at menopause
	• As required if under treatment for osteoporosis
Skin cancer	• Age twenty through forty, every three years
	• After age forty, every year—especially if at high risk
Electrocardiogram	• Establish baseline in late thirties
	• Before embarking on strenuous exercise program
Dental cleaning	• Twice a year
	• For smokers, also screen for oral cancer
Eye exam	• After age forty, every three years; After age sixty-five, annually
	• Should include screen for glaucoma
AIDS test	• Every six months for those at high risk (for example, sexually active people who are not in monogamous relationships, health-care workers, those intimate with IV drug user)
Immunizations	• Discuss your immunization history with your physician.
	• Inquire specifically about: tetanus-diphtheria booster, measles, rubella, pneumonia, influenza, hepatitis B.

STRATEGY 1: MAINTAIN A HEALTHY WEIGHT

The human body is a remarkably efficient machine, and nowhere is this more evident than in our ability to store fat. We inherited this mixed blessing from our ancient ancestors who needed to keep their body-fat level high in case the next hunt for food was unsuccessful. Although you probably don't have to worry about where your next meal is coming from, your body is still programmed to protect you from starvation.

I call this evolutionary adaptation a mixed blessing because, given our abundance of food, it can interfere with maintaining a healthy weight. Nevertheless, there are times we still need its protection. For example, when stricken with disease or severe injury, we can call upon fat stores to provide the energy we need for recovery. And our built-in resistance to losing weight is a first line of defense against the dangerous effects of chronic dieting and eating disorders (see chapter 5).

Maintaining a *healthy* weight is achieving a balance—not too heavy, not too thin. If you are too thin, you may be suffering from an eating disorder that, left untreated, can be fatal (see chapter 5). Being too thin also interferes with estrogen production. For adolescents and young adults, that means peak bone mass will be compromised and the risk for osteoporosis thereby increased. Women who are too thin during their childbearing years may have problems related to fertility. In older women, loss of body fat may affect bone density. Older women who do not have enough body fat also are more vulnerable to bone fractures resulting from falls.

The health consequences of obesity are equally, if not more, devastating (see chapter 2). Health experts agree that obesity has become epidemic in this country, especially among women. Approximately 150,000 women die each year from diseases directly related to obesity—heart disease, diabetes and some cancers. Obesity also contributes to hypertension, high cholesterol, osteoarthritis, immune dysfunction and infertility—not to mention its psychological toll resulting from our culture's emphasis on being thin.

What Is Your Healthy Weight?

As we've learned more about the relationship between weight and health, we've also discovered that determining "healthy weight" involves more than checking a standardized table. In fact, height-weight tables can't begin to account for the many variables that exist from person to person. So as a first step, I suggest you look at not one but three, perhaps four, measurements: height for weight, body mass index (BMI), waist-hip ratio (WHR) and percentage of body fat. It may sound complicated, but it's really not.

Height for Weight: There is some controversy over exactly which of several height-weight tables is most useful. I prefer the table included in the latest version of the Dietary Guidelines for Americans.

Height (without shoes)	Weight Range (all adults)
(feet, inches)	(pounds)
4'10"	91–119
4'11"	94–124
5'0"	97–128
5'1"	101–132
5'2"	104–137
5'3"	107–141
5'4"	111–146
5'5"	114–150
5'6"	118–155
5'7"	121–160
5'8"	125–164
5'9"	129–169
5'10"	132–174
5'11"	136–179
6'0"	140–184
6'1"	144–189
6'2"	148–195

The desirable weight for women is generally at the lower end of the range.

Earlier height-weight tables included two age ranges, nineteen to thirty-four and thirty-five and older, and allowed for some weight gain as you aged. For example, a five-foot-five-inch woman might weigh 114 at age nineteen and 126 at age thirty-five. Today, experts generally agree that you should try to avoid gaining weight as you age. The typical ten- to fifteen-pound gain between early adulthood and middle age should act as an early warning to make some lifestyle changes.

Body mass index (BMI): Researchers are always looking for better ways to measure obesity and to predict associated health risks. These days, when you go for a physical, you are likely to have your body mass index (BMI) calculated. BMI is a ratio based on the *relationship* between height and weight and is considered a relatively accurate measurement of obesity. You can determine your BMI by multiplying your weight in pounds by 700 and dividing the result by the square of your height in inches (see chapter 2 for a BMI chart).

As with height-weight tables, there is some controversy over what constitutes a healthy BMI. Recent research that was widely reported in the press might lead you to believe that a BMI over 19 puts you at a considerable health risk, especially for heart disease. In fact, a BMI between 19 and 25 is considered relatively healthy, if you don't have any extenuating health problems putting you at risk for diabetes or heart disease. Your risk of premature death increases markedly, however, with a BMI over 27. A BMI under 19 is also cause for concern. The graph below combines the current height-weight table with BMIs to illustrate general healthy weight, moderately overweight and severely overweight ranges.

ARE YOU OVERWEIGHT?

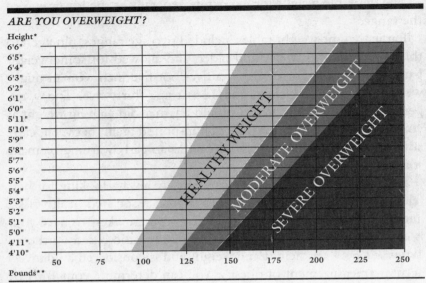

*Without shoes.

**Without clothes. The higher weights apply to people with more muscle and bone, such as many men.

Source: *Report of the Dietary Guidelines Advisory Committee on the Dietary Guidelines for Americans, 1995*, pages 23–24.

A weakness of both height-weight tables and BMI is that neither will apply if you have large bones or are very muscular. According to both measures, you probably would be classified as "overweight," when in fact you are likely to be lean and at a healthy weight.

Waist-Hip Ratio (WHR): Another measurement used to predict health risk from obesity is waist-hip ratio. WHR identifies proportion of upper-body fat to lower-body fat. As I indicated earlier, researchers have determined that upper-body fat (apple-shaped body) is associated with a greater health risk than lower-body fat (pear-shaped body). To determine your WHR, divide your waist measurement (at the area of smallest girth above your navel) by your hip measurement (at the largest horizontal girth between your waist and thighs). If your WHR is greater than 0.8, you are at increased risk, especially for heart disease.

Some researchers believe you don't have to calculate WHR to assess your risk from upper-body fat. A waist measurement of thirty-one inches or more may be enough to signal concern. And like height-weight tables and BMI, WHR has its drawbacks. If you are very thin or very overweight, it is not such a reliable indicator of risk.

Percentage of Body Fat: A healthy weight isn't just a low number on the height-weight chart, a good BMI and a good WHR. It's also a healthy balance between body fat and muscle or lean body mass. The consensus is that for optimal health women should have 19 percent to 30 percent body fat depending on age. As you get older, you will lose muscle and gain fat—even though your weight may stay the same.

Unfortunately, body fat is not easy to measure. If you want to determine yours, talk to your physician, a nutrition professional or a professional trainer about a bioelectric impedance test or underwater weighing. An easier, less expensive alternative, though not as accurate, is a skin-fold test using special calipers. Even easier is looking in the mirror. If, despite good BMI and WHR numbers, you look "flabby," chances are you have more body fat than is healthy and need to build lean body mass.

After you've checked all these numbers, you'll have a fairly good idea if your current weight is healthy. But there are still some other important variables to consider, including your age, cholesterol levels, blood pressure and blood glucose level, your medical history, and your family history. The more risk factors you identify, the more conscientious you need to be about your weight. If, however, your weight, BMI and WHR are somewhat high, and you are otherwise "metabolically healthy," you needn't be overly concerned about shedding some pounds immediately. Just be aware of the situation and keep an eye on things.

Assessing Your Weight
Healthy weight is more than a number on the scale. All these factors contribute to your weight profile. Discuss the details with your doctor or a nutrition professional.

The "Numbers"	Your Personal Risk Factors	Your Family History
Height-Weight Table	◆ Age	
Weight range considered	◆ Gender	
safe for height	◆ Percent body fat	
Body Mass Index (BMI)	◆ Total cholesterol	
Degree of health risk	◆ LDL cholesterol	
associated with height-	◆ HDL cholesterol	
weight ratio	◆ Triglycerides	
Waist-Hip Ratio (WHR)	◆ Blood pressure	
Degree of health risk	◆ Blood sugar	
associated with	◆ Medical history	
location of body fat		

Setting Healthy Weight Goals

After you look at all the numbers, consider your personal risk factors and review your family history, you may decide to try to lose some weight. Although heredity plays an important role in determining the upper and lower limits of your weight, you can do a lot to control how your weight fluctuates within that range. But when you set a weight goal for yourself, be realistic. For example, what is the least you've weighed as an adult and have been able to maintain for at least a year (without constantly dieting)?

Set an initial, reasonable goal, which may not be the total amount of weight you'd eventually like to lose. Remember that losing even 5 percent to 10 percent of your current weight will result in major health benefits. After you achieve that loss and maintain it for six to twelve months, reassess your situation. Recalculate your BMI and WHR and take another look at your personal risk factors. If your weight is still higher than "desirable" and if your risk factors still put you at risk, reward yourself for progress so far and set a new weight-loss goal of 5 percent to 10 percent of your current weight or ten to fifteen pounds. Keep repeating this incremental pattern until you achieve a healthy weight. This slow, steady approach will help keep your spirits up, enhance your sense of control and make it easier to maintain your weight loss.

Once you've set your goal, you need to calculate how many calories you should eat each day and still achieve that goal. Notice I say "should eat," not "are allowed to eat." That's because if you eat too few calories, you might not lose weight. Your body may think it's starving and that survival mechanism I talked about earlier will kick in. Your metabolism will slow down and your body will conserve fat— exactly the opposite of what you are trying to achieve. Here is an easy rule of thumb for calculating the number of calories you need:

1. Multiply what you weigh now by 15 if you are moderately active, or 13 if you are sedentary. The number you get represents the average number of calories you need each day to maintain your current weight. For example, a moderately active 150-pound woman uses about 2,250 calories a day (150 x 15 = 2,250).

2. To determine an appropriate target for weight loss, subtract 20 percent of your maintenance calories. If your daily maintenance level is 2,250 calories, your weight loss level is 1,800 calories (2,250 x .2 = 450; 2,250 − 450 = 1,800). You can achieve this calorie deficit by eating fewer calories or by burning more calories through exercising—or by a combination of both. Strategy 2 gives you more information on increasing physical activity.

Keep in mind that for safety and long-term maintenance, you should aim to lose only one-half pound to one pound a week. Reducing your daily calorie intake by 500 per day will result in a loss of about 1 pound per week (500 calories x 7 days = 3,500 calories = one pound). But don't drop under 1,200 calories per day. Below that number, your body tends to fight back by lowering your metabolism and thwarting your weight-loss efforts. If you are trying to maintain your weight, not lose weight, calculate your maintenance calories (step 1) and stop there. A nutrition professional can be very helpful in refining these goals for you so that they are truly tailor-made.

Divide your calorie budget into a balanced, realistic plan including at least three meals a day plus snacks or, even better, six mini-meals. About 50 percent to 55 percent of your calories should come from carbohydrates, 15 percent to 20 percent from protein and no more than 30 percent from fat. Use the Food Guide Pyramid and the food label (see chapter 4) to help you plan meals, select foods and choose portions that will give you the most nutrition along with the best taste and greatest satisfaction. Strategy 3 gives you more information on designing a healthy eating plan that emphasizes carbohydrate foods like fruit, vegetables and grains.

Remember, a deprivation diet won't work. Yes, you are trying to lose weight but you are also working on building lifelong healthy eating habits. Your food should taste good and leave you feeling satisfied. Those two aspects of your new approach to eating are just as important to your physical and psychological health as good nutrition.

If you have become used to following a restrictive diet, it may take you awhile to get out of that habit. For example, you may be uncomfortable eating a number of small meals throughout the day. But keep in mind that doing so is one way to keep hunger to a minimum. When you feel hungry, you are more likely to binge. Eating a series of small meals also keeps your metabolism on an even keel, keeps blood sugar stable and may enable the body to use nutrients more efficiently.

If you have never paid much attention to what you eat and when you eat, keep a food diary. People who have reached a healthy weight and have maintained it say that logging their food—and their exercise, too—was the single most important thing they did to achieve success. Research shows that, when asked to recall, most people underestimate their food intake and overestimate their exercise. But when you keep an honest log in real time, the facts are there in black and white.

Some people include in each log entry the time of day, what they are doing besides eating (driving? watching TV?) and a note on their mood. When you review your diary, this information can help you analyze your "food triggers"—the people, places and things that may send you to the cookie jar to cope. Certainly, one dimension of reaching and maintaining a healthy weight is recognizing and defusing these triggers. If emotional trouble persists, consider seeing a counselor to get to the root of it. Your doctor, clergy person or nutrition professional can give you a referral.

Whether you are trying to lose weight or overcome an eating disorder that has left you dangerously thin, remember that reaching and maintaining a healthy weight is a process. For many women, this process can be very challenging work. For some, it is a matter of life and death. Above all, be kind to yourself. Your healthy weight is not society's decision, your family's decision or your friends' decision. It is 100 percent your decision based on your health profile and the choices you make.

Tips

◆ Serve your meals on smaller plates. Doing so will help you adjust to smaller portions without feeling deprived.

◆ In a restaurant, if portions are too large, ask for a take-out package before you begin eating. Pack up half the meal for tomorrow.

◆ Buy the smallest-size packages of snacks and cookies. Research shows that we eat more when we see those big bags and boxes.

◆ Eat slowly and enjoy your food. Remember it takes twenty minutes for your brain to tell your stomach you are full.

◆ Don't skip breakfast. It jump-starts your metabolism for the day.

◆ Think quality not quantity when it comes to indulging yourself. For example, buy super-rich chocolate and enjoy a small but intense taste of it now and then.

◆ One hundred extra calories a day—about the amount in a glass of wine—add up to 700 calories a week, equal to a ten-pound weight gain in one year!

◆ Cook once, but eat twice or more. For example, roast a chicken and use it all week—in stir-fries, sandwiches, salads, soups and stews.

◆ Encourage your children to be physically active. Obese children and adolescents have up to an 80 percent chance of becoming obese adults.

◆ Don't put your family on a diet. Instead, involve them in your effort to eat healthier.

How to Choose a Weight-Loss Program

If you decide to try a commercial weight-loss program, investigate your options carefully. Naturally, you'll want a safe, reasonably priced program with features that will meet your unique needs. Here are some questions to consider:

- **Are you ready to commit to losing weight and keeping it off?** Try to focus on health rather than appearance. You'll be more successful in the long run.
- **Does the program you are considering include ongoing weight-maintenance support?** Quick-fix weight-loss programs won't give you long-term results. Learning how to maintain your weight by changing eating and other lifestyle behaviors is the key to lifelong health benefits.
- **Does the program encourage physical activity?** Exercise not only promotes weight loss; it also helps you maintain a healthy weight. A good program advocates physical activity and shows you how to increase your level of exercise gradually and safely.
- **What does the program suggest as your goal weight and how long will it take you to reach it?** Your goal weight should be realistic and based on your personal and family weight history—not just height and weight charts. Remember even a ten-pound weight loss will have positive health benefits. The slower you lose weight, the more likely you are to keep it off. A one-half- to one-pound loss per week is a safe goal. (You may lose weight more rapidly at first, but this loss is mostly water.) If you plan to lose more than twenty pounds, if you have any health problems or if you take medication on a regular basis, consult your doctor before starting a weight-loss plan.
- **What is the program format?** If you need a lot of social support, you might want to join a self-help-style group. If you are enthusiastic about exercise, investigate programs offered by health clubs. If you need a great deal of structure, look for a

group that will give you a specific step-by-step plan tailored to your needs. If you don't respond well to a group, consider individual counseling with a nutrition professional.

◆ **Does the program suit your lifestyle?** If you travel a lot or dine out often, you'll want a program that is flexible and teaches you how to incorporate healthy eating into your schedule.

◆ **Does the program exclude any foods or rely on megadoses of any food or nutrient?** If so, stop right there. No safe weight-loss or weight-management plan will exclude or overemphasize any one food or nutrient. A sensible plan also will leave some room for an occasional splurge. Balance, variety and moderation should be your watchwords. If a program includes its own prepackaged foods, ask for samples and make sure the products suit your taste before you sign up. If you don't like the food, you won't stick with the program. In any program, your daily calorie level should not fall below 1,200 calories.

◆ **Do you understand program fees?** Advertised fees may not reflect *total* costs. Items like videos and audiotapes may cost extra. If the program includes prepackaged foods, figure that cost into your assessment. If you pay a flat fee, be sure you know how much time you are actually buying versus how much time you think you'll need.

◆ **What is the program's track record?** Any program you are considering should be willing to tell you:

  ◆ The percentage of participants who achieve various degrees of weight loss
  ◆ The amount of weight loss typically maintained for a year or more
  ◆ The percentage of participants who experience adverse effects

◆ **How are program counselors trained in weight loss and weight maintenance?** Protect your health—and your investment—by asking for background information on how staffers are trained and supervised. The program should have a nutrition professional available to answer counselors' questions.

How to Find a Nutrition Professional

Rather than joining a structured weight loss or maintenance program, you may prefer to work one-on-one with a nutrition professional. You will find people who call themselves nutritionists with all kinds of so-called credentials. Some may sound impressive but could mean absolutely nothing. Look for the credential R.D., which stands for "registered dietitian." At a minimum, R.D.'s have earned an undergraduate degree and served an internship in some aspect of nutrition. Many hold graduate degrees as well. In addition, all registered dietitians must pass a rigorous credentialing examination and pursue continuing education in order to keep their credentials current. To help protect consumers, some states also license registered dietitians, so you might see the credential L.D. along with R.D.

Before your first visit, it is likely that a registered dietitian will ask you to keep a food diary for at least three days, including one weekend day. This record will help your R.D. understand your eating habits and spot any nutritional deficiencies. You also might be asked to provide some medical information—such as your cholesterol level and blood pressure.

At your first visit, your dietitian will weigh you and is likely to calculate your body mass index (BMI) and waist-hip (WHR) ratio. He or she also might use skin calipers to estimate your body fat-to-lean ratio. (This procedure is painless.) Your dietitian will review your medical history, lifestyle, activity level, shopping and eating habits, family medical history, and, of course, your goals. Based on all this information, your R.D. will help you make a plan for weight loss or weight maintenance and will follow your progress over an agreed-upon period of time, making adjustments as needed.

The initial visit with a registered dietitian (about an hour) will cost $50 to $100. Follow-up visits may be less. Some insurance plans cover these costs if you are referred by your physician for a medical necessity. To find an R.D. in your area, ask your doctor or call the American Dietetic Association's National Nutrition Network, (800) 366-1655.

Weight-Loss Drugs: The Facts

Weight-loss drugs like Redux and fen-phen, which change levels of the brain chemicals that influence appetite, are among the best medical discoveries to hit the market in years—but not for the reasons you may think. Their value is not in their ability to help you shed a fast ten or twenty pounds. Rather, these drugs are important because they signal a fundamental change in the way we look at obesity.

For a long time, obesity was considered a matter of weak willpower or poor character. Now we know it is a biologically based chronic condition that requires lifelong treatment. Medication is part of the treatment for chronic conditions like diabetes and hypertension. Why not for obesity as well?

In fact, the Food and Drug Administration (FDA) has approved Redux (dexfenfluramine) and fen-phen (fenfluramine/Pondimin and phentermine/Ionamin) for use *only* by people whose weight is a health hazard. Unfortunately, however, almost anyone who tries hard enough can get a prescription. It's not surprising that sales of Redux alone total about $20 million a month. People have been known to travel across the country to clinics where the drugs are easy to come by. There have been reports of people wearing ankle weights to tip the scales upward and boost their chances of getting a prescription. One doctor is even dispensing prescriptions from his home page on the Internet.

These drugs are attractive because, unlike the amphetamine-based weight-loss medications of the 1950s and 1960s, they are not addictive. And they can help many people, though not all, shed pounds. But they are clearly not intended for casual use. Their effect is generally short-term—usually six to twelve months—and most people begin regaining the weight they have lost as soon as they stop taking the pills.

Both Redux and fen-phen also have side effects ranging from annoying but harmless dry mouth to rare but potentially fatal pulmonary hypertension (high blood pressure in the artery to the lungs). There also is some evidence from animal studies that high doses of either drug can alter brain chemistry. After reviewing twenty studies spanning thirty years, the National Task Force on the Prevention and Treatment of Obesity concluded that despite their short-term effectiveness, not enough is known about the safety and effectiveness of these drugs beyond one year of use. Consequently, the task force cautioned against their long-term use—even for the chronically obese.

So whether you are medically obese or just thinking about jump-starting a weight-loss program with a few months of Redux or fen-phen, please think again. You will probably lose weight, but without exercise you won't build muscle mass or improve your cardiovascular fitness. And after you stop the medication, you are likely to regain what you lost.

At least two commercial weight-loss plans are making Redux and fen-phen available to their clients through in-house or affiliated doctors. But don't get involved in a program like this until you consult your *own* physician, especially if you are already taking antidepressant medication or if you have heart disease.

There are several more weight-loss drugs in development. In addition, obesity researchers recently discovered the UCP2 gene, which activates the protein that seems to be responsible for burning calories as body heat rather than storing them as fat. A drug to "turn on" this gene may be available in as little as five years.

Benefits of Maintaining a Healthy Weight by Life Stage

Children
- ◆ Helps prevent adult obesity.
- ◆ Helps keep cholesterol and triglycerides at healthy levels.

Adolescents and young women
- ◆ Helps prevent adult obesity.
- ◆ Boosts self-esteem.
- ◆ Promotes bone density and achievement of peak bone mass.
- ◆ Promotes lifelong heart health.
- ◆ May make breast cancer easier to detect.
- ◆ Helps prevent hypertension, high cholesterol and diabetes.
- ◆ Lowers risk of arthritis in later life.

Premenopausal women
- ◆ Enhances fertility.
- ◆ Protects against heart disease, diabetes and some cancers.
- ◆ May make breast cancer easier to detect.
- ◆ Helps prevent gallbladder disease.

Postmenopausal women
- ◆ Helps prevent "middle-age spread"—potentially risky upper-body weight.
- ◆ Protects against heart disease, diabetes and some cancers (including breast cancer).

Older women
- ◆ Protects against loss of bone density; cushions bones from fracture.
- ◆ Protects against heart disease, diabetes and some cancers.
- ◆ Will help ameliorate body wasting in case of severe illness.

Pregnant and lactating women (Check with your doctor before starting any weight-loss plan.)
- ◆ Affects fetal growth; reduces risk of preterm birth and infant mortality.
- ◆ Makes childbirth easier/safer.
- ◆ Helps prevent future maternal obesity.
- ◆ Helps ensure volume and quality of breast milk.

Points to Remember

About your weight:

◆ Healthy weight is more than a number on a scale or a chart. It depends on variables such as your personal risk factors and family history.

◆ Even a small weight loss can have significant health benefits.

◆ If you want to lose weight, set a realistic initial goal of 5 to 10 percent of your current weight or ten to fifteen pounds.

STRATEGY 2: ENJOY PHYSICAL ACTIVITY

Burning fat and calories through exercise is an important part of maintaining a healthy weight. The latest version of the Dietary Guidelines for Americans encourages balancing food intake with physical activity. But regular physical activity does a lot more than keep extra pounds in check.

In fact, some scientists believe that many of the effects we associate with getting older are not so much the result of aging as they are of inactivity. Between ages twenty and thirty, your body strength is at its peak. Starting around age forty, slow, subtle changes begin. You start to lose lean body mass, muscle tone and stamina, and you take in less oxygen. But if you follow a regular exercise program, you can counteract this process and maintain a high level of fitness.

Recent research suggests that a sedentary person—young or old—has the same risk of dying prematurely as a person who smokes a pack of cigarettes a day. In fact, experts suggest that lack of physical activity may be implicated in as many as 250,000 deaths each year. Yet, despite a growing body of overwhelming evidence on the dangers of being a couch potato, only about 20 percent of adults engage in regular physical activity of any intensity. And among overweight adults, more than a third don't participate in any physical activity.

A "Fountain of Youth"

While there is no magic formula to fitness, we do know that exercise is a key component in a healthy lifestyle. I urge you to take a closer look at how much exercise you get, especially after I tell you some more about how physical activity comes closer than anything we know to a fountain of youth (see also chapter 2). Some experts maintain that exercise is especially vital to women of all ages because the risk for so many of the diseases we're vulnerable to can be lowered by getting rid of body fat.

Consider heart disease and stroke. Although most of the research on cardiovascular disease and exercise has been done on men, recent studies are showing that exercise is good for women's cardiovascular health, too. Exercise helps reduce the risk of heart disease and stroke by strengthening the heart muscle, lowering blood pressure, raising protective HDL cholesterol and lowering damaging LDL cholesterol, reducing the risk for developing blood clots and diabetes, and helping to control weight gain.

For older people who are at a healthy weight, regular exercise preserves muscle tissue and helps prevent body fat from accumulating in the abdominal area, where it poses a risk for heart disease and perhaps for breast disease.

The link between exercise and colon cancer is fairly well established, and there is reason to believe exercise may protect against breast cancer in premenopausal woman by lengthening the menstrual cycle and thus cutting down on the body's exposure to estrogen. Reducing body fat through exercise also may help to prevent breast cancer, especially among postmenopausal women, because fat cells produce a type of estrogen.

In the prevention and treatment of osteoporosis, exercise is critical for building bone mass early in life and for preventing bone loss in the later years. Exercise also builds flexibility, strength and coordination—all of which can help older women avoid the falls that lead to hip fracture and other injuries. Recent research also shows that regular physical activity helps people with osteoarthritis go about their daily lives with more flexibility and less pain.

Physical activity helps to prevent and treat type 2 diabetes by increasing the body's sensitivity to insulin, which lowers blood sugar. Regular exercise also helps maintain a healthy body weight not only by burning calories and fat, but also by building muscle tissue. The more muscle you have, the more calories your body burns, even when you are resting. And some research indicates that exercise is the most effective way to keep weight off after you've lost it.

Physical activity also increases the circulation of immune cells. Increasingly, research is showing that the body's ability to fight infections and malignant cells is tied to an immune system boosted by regular exercise. Physical activity has long been known as an antidote for depression; recent research suggests it also can play a role in improving sleep, especially in older people who often battle insomnia. Regular exercise also may help to preserve memory and reaction time in older people.

If all these reasons aren't enough to motivate you to up your level of physical activity, consider that exercise just plain makes you feel good. People who exercise regularly just for pleasure say it is a great way to develop positive feelings about your body. And the good news is that moderate exercisers feel just as good about themselves as people who exercise a lot. In addition, the calming brain chemicals known as endorphins increase with exercise. Scientists have linked endorphins with the ability to tolerate pain, control appetite and reduce tension and anxiety. It may be that people who exercise regularly, need less activity to feel the effect of endorphins. The calming chemicals may last longer in the bloodstreams of regular exercisers as well.

Finally, some research suggests that women who work out on a regular basis feel better about themselves, perhaps because they develop a sense of mastery that enhances self-esteem.

How Active Are You?

Before you continue to read this chapter, take a minute to see how active you are.

If you . . .	You are . . .
☐ Get no exercise.	Sedentary
☐ Use stairs and walk briskly; do gardening, housework and/or exercise 3–5 times per week for 20–30 minutes.	Moderately active
☐ Use stairs and walk briskly; exercise 3–5 times per week for 60 minutes a session.	Active
☐ Use stairs and walk briskly; exercise 3–5 times per week for 90 minutes a session (or for more than 60 minutes daily); engage in other daily physical activity; are a recreational athlete.	Very active
☐ Use stairs and walk briskly; exercise 5 or more times per week for 120 minutes (daily or more than once for 90 minutes); engage in other daily physical activity; are a professional athlete.	Extremely active

Physical Activity vs. Exercise: Is There a Difference?

Yes—and no. Physical activity includes what we traditionally think of as exercise (for example, using the stationary bike or the treadmill), but it also encompasses everyday activities like climbing stairs, doing housework, playing with the children and gardening. We now know that to be beneficial, physical activity need not be the intense, vigorous, "no pain–no gain" variety.

150 Calories—Gone!

Washing/waxing the car	45–60 minutes
Washing windows or floors	45–60 minutes
Playing volleyball	45 minutes
Gardening	30–45 minutes
Walking 1 3/4 miles in . . .	35 minutes
Shooting hoops	30 minutes
Bicycling 5 miles in . . .	30 minutes
Dancing fast	30 minutes
Raking leaves	30 minutes
Walking 2 miles in . . .	30 minutes
Water aerobics	30 minutes
Swimming laps	20 minutes
Bicycling 4 miles in . . .	15 minutes
Jumping rope	15 minutes
Shoveling snow	15 minutes
Stair walking	15 minutes

In early 1995, the Centers for Disease Control and the American College of Sports Medicine recommended that to increase longevity and reduce disease risk we should accumulate thirty minutes or more of moderate-intensity physical activity on most, preferably all, days of the week. The Dietary Guidelines and the Surgeon General's recent report, *Physical Activity and Health,* support this recommendation. For most healthy adults, moderate physical activity is the equivalent of brisk walking at three to four miles an hour. While older guidelines recommended twenty to sixty continuous minutes of intense exercise, the new guideline stresses that we can *accumulate* thirty minutes of daily activity—ideally enough to expend about 150 to 200 calories a day.

As in the study of diet and disease, there are controversies in exercise research, too. You have probably read about studies that challenge the effectiveness of this latest guideline. For example, a Harvard study suggested that longevity is fostered only by intense, not moderate, exercise. Part of the confusion here, acknowledged by the Harvard researchers, has to do with semantics—one person's idea of intense may be someone else's definition of moderate. Thus, study participants may not have been consistent in reporting the true nature of their exercise.

So where does that leave you? Here is the bottom line on the exercise controversy: A little exercise is better than none, but more is even better. In fact, the most dramatic positive effects occur in people who go from being unfit to moderately fit. Even in the unlikely event that moderate exercise does nothing to promote longevity and help prevent disease, it still will enhance quality of life by helping with weight control, making it easier to perform daily tasks as you age and enhancing psychological well-being.

If you are already physically active, take it up a notch or two (but don't overdo it!). You'll reap even more benefits. Think about a weight-training program or regular aerobic exercise to give your heart and lungs a real workout. If you are fairly inactive, start by making small changes like taking the stairs instead of the elevator and parking farther away from your destination so you have to do some walking. I know you've probably heard advice like this a million times. But it really can make a difference. Small changes help to shape your attitude toward fitness and to ease you into making physical activity a routine part of your life. And when you break thirty minutes of physical activity into three ten-minute segments, it's not so hard to work exercise into a busy day.

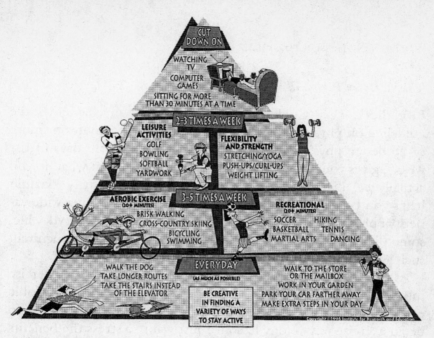

CUT DOWN ON
WATCHING TV
COMPUTER GAMES
SITTING FOR MORE THAN 30 MINUTES AT A TIME

2-3 TIMES A WEEK

LEISURE ACTIVITIES
GOLF
BOWLING
SOFTBALL
YARDWORK

FLEXIBILITY AND STRENGTH
STRETCHING/YOGA
PUSH-UPS/CURL-UPS
WEIGHT LIFTING

3-5 TIMES A WEEK

AEROBIC EXERCISE (20+ MINUTES)
BRISK WALKING
CROSS-COUNTRY SKIING
BICYCLING
SWIMMING

RECREATIONAL (20+ MINUTES)
SOCCER   HIKING
BASKETBALL TENNIS
MARTIAL ARTS DANCING

EVERYDAY
(AS MUCH AS POSSIBLE)

WALK THE DOG
TAKE LONGER ROUTES
TAKE THE STAIRS INSTEAD OF THE ELEVATOR

BE CREATIVE IN FINDING A VARIETY OF WAYS TO STAY ACTIVE

WALK TO THE STORE OR THE MAILBOX
WORK IN YOUR GARDEN
PARK YOUR CAR FARTHER AWAY
MAKE EXTRA STEPS IN YOUR DAY

Copyright ©1996 Institute for Research and Education

If you are inactive, increase activities from the base of the pyramid by

- Taking the stairs instead of the elevator
- Making extra trips around the house or yard
- Stretching while standing on line

If you are somewhat active, use the middle of the pyramid to

- Find activities you enjoy
- Schedule activities into your day
- Set realistic goals and stick to them

If you are active, use the middle of the pyramid to

- Change your routine if you start to get bored
- Explore new activities

The Activity Pyramid

Like the Dietary Guidelines we talked about in chapter 4, the guideline on physical activity—accumulate thirty minutes or more of moderate physical activity on most, preferably all, days of the week—gives you some basic, general information. But what do you actually *do?* Like the Food Guide Pyramid, the Activity Pyramid helps you balance your exercise and make choices from a wide variety of physical activities—some that are part of your everyday life, some that are leisure activities and some that are more structured, such as workouts.

As you move up the pyramid and incorporate more exercise into your life, you'll want to strike a balance between aerobic exercise, strength training and stretching. This isn't going to be an exercise physiology lesson. I just want to stress the benefits of all three types of activity so that you can use them effectively. Like the foods in your diet, different activities have different benefits.

What's Your Target Heart Rate?

Your target heart rate or training zone is between 50 percent and 75 percent of your maximum heart rate (beats per minute) for your age. Here's how to calculate yours:

1. Subtract your age from 220.
2. Multiply the result by 75 percent (0.75) and then by 50% (0.5).

The first figure is the top of your training zone, and the second is the bottom. As you become more fit, you'll have to work harder to reach your maximum rate.

Age (years)	Target Heart Rate Zone (beats per minute)
20	100–150
25	98–146
30	95–142
35	93–138
40	90–135
45	88–131
50	85–127
55	83–123
60	80–120
65	78–116
70	75–113

Here is how to check if you are within your target heart zone.

1. While exercising, take your pulse by placing your first two fingers lightly on your neck just to either side of your Adam's apple, or on the inside of your wrist just below the base of your thumb.
2. Count your pulse for ten seconds and multiply by six to get beats per minute (sixty seconds).

If it's not convenient to check your heart rate—for example, if you're walking briskly and pumping your arms—use the "out of breath" test. You are at or close to your maximum heart rate if you have enough breath to speak, but just barely, as you are exercising.

◆ **Aerobic exercise,** or cardiovascular exercise, keeps your heart and lungs vigorous. Full benefit to your circulatory system comes with exercising enough to raise your heartbeat to your target heart rate zone (see sidebar What's Your Target Heart Rate, pages 186–187) for twenty to thirty minutes, three to five times a week. As your body adapts, you won't have to work so hard to reach your target heart rate. If your heart rate drops, you'll have to pick up the intensity to boost it back into the training zone. In addition to conditioning your heart and lungs, intense aerobic exercise also burns calories and fat. Even after you stop exercising, your metabolism can stay revved up for as much as an hour. Weight-bearing aerobic exercise with an impact, like walking, step aerobics and jumping rope, also helps to build bones.

The best all-around aerobic exercises are cross-country skiing, rowing and swimming because they involve all the major muscle groups of the upper and lower body. Other good aerobic activities are brisk walking, jogging, cycling, skating, water or step aerobics, jumping rope, playing vigorous racquet sports, and working out on a treadmill, exercise bike or step machine.

◆ **Strength training** builds and tones muscle. Although aerobic exercise builds some muscles, lifting weights or working out on resistance machines is a much more targeted approach. Building muscle is key to maintaining a healthy weight. Even though minute for minute, aerobic exercise burns more calories than strength training, the new muscle tissue you build with strength training burns 25 percent more calories than any fat tissue it replaces—even when you are sitting still or sleeping. And although you may weigh more as you build muscle, because muscle by volume weighs more than fat, you will trim down in size, because muscle takes up less space than fat. Your metabolic rate also stays elevated for a while after strength training.

Strength training also helps build bones by stimulating the muscles attached to them. It also contributes to flexibility and balance, which are especially important for preventing falls among older people. If you have been sedentary for quite a while, you might want to do some training with weights before you try any aerobic exercise. It will improve your balance and your strength, making injury less likely.

◆ **Stretching** promotes flexibility and protects against injury. Over time, stretching lengthens muscles and strengthens ligaments and tendons. The result is less stiffness, a greater range of motion and relief from muscle tension. Both yoga and tai chi are forms of stretching.

As with any good thing, there is such a thing as too much. Moderation is as important in physical activity as it is in diet. In fact, beyond a certain point, exercise begins to have the reverse of its positive effects. In chapter 5, we talked about the physical effects of severe stress like injury or burns. Extreme exercise can cause some of the same reactions, including a decline in immunity. In addition, too much exercise can interrupt your menstrual cycle, interfere with fertility, cause bone loss, create a constant state of fatigue and trigger eating disorders.

Tips

◆ If you are planning to start a program of aerobic exercise, begin with some weight training to build up your strength.

◆ Muscle burns more calories than fat. The more muscle tissue you have, the more calories you will burn—even sitting still or sleeping.

◆ The more active you are, the more calories you can eat while still maintaining a healthy weight.

◆ Make your own "free weights." Use full soup cans or milk jugs filled with water or sand for hand weights. For leg weights, drape socks filled with beans over your ankles.

◆ You'll know you're lifting the right amount of weight if you can do only eight to twelve repetitions before your muscles are tired.

◆ Toning exercises won't help you lose weight in one particular area of your body. The only way to lose fat is to build muscle and burn off calories.

◆ It's safe to do aerobic exercise every day, but let your muscles rest one day between strength-training sessions—or do upper-body work one day followed by lower-body work the next day.

◆ The next time you have to run to answer the phone, carry a two-year-old around the mall or dash through an airport to catch a plane, think of it as an aerobic opportunity.

◆ Between ages thirty and eighty, you lost about 40 percent of your muscle mass and 30 percent of your strength. Much of this loss can be prevented or even reversed with strength training. And you're never too old to start!

◆ If you walk at 140 steps per minute, you're moving at a rate of four miles per hour.

◆ Running creates a force equal to 2.5 times your body weight. Low-impact exercise—like brisk walking—reduces the risk of discomfort and injury.

◆ Encourage your children and grandchildren to enjoy more physical activity. During the 1990s, daily attendance in physical education classes among high school students declined from 42 percent to 25 percent.

◆ If it isn't safe or convenient to walk in your neighborhood, try walking briskly through your local mall early in the morning before the crowds arrive.

◆ The most important piece of exercise equipment you can buy is a good pair of multipurpose athletic shoes. Go to a reputable store and explain your needs to a well-trained sales consultant. Bargain shoes can be a costly mistake!

◆ Bicycling isn't considered as good a weight-bearing activity as walking for building bone because when you're seated you're not supporting all of your body weight. To boost the bone-building ability of biking, cycle at a higher tension. That will place more stress on your muscles and stimulate your bones.

◆ Morning, noon or night: When is the best time to work out? There are reasons to support each one, but the bottom line is: When will you *really do it*?

Setting Your Physical Activity Goals

Before you start any kind of rigorous exercise program, check with your physician. If you are fairly sedentary now, start with the basic guideline: thirty minutes of moderate exercise accumulated throughout the day. To build bone and muscle and boost overall strength, consider adding two or three strength-training sessions a week. You don't have to buy a lot of fancy equipment or join a health club. When you are ready, you may want to learn simple weight-lifting techniques from a video or in a few sessions with a personal trainer. A good video or a trainer should explain lifting techniques as well as some stretches for the muscles you've worked. To avoid injury, always warm up for a couple of minutes by doing something simple like marching in place or jumping jacks.

Strength training will help you maintain a healthy weight by building calorie-burning muscle. You may want to add some aerobic exercise for your heart health. Aerobic exercise will also help with weight management and bone building. Work up to three weekly aerobic sessions—brisk walking, perhaps—and work out for twenty minutes at your maximum heart rate. After you get hooked on exercise, you may want to join a health club.

Like healthy eating, enjoying physical activity is a lifelong pursuit. The benefits are continuous but only as long as you stick with a regular plan. As hard as you try, though, you probably won't be able to keep a rigid schedule. But feeling guilty about not exercising doesn't work any better than feeling guilty about that piece of chocolate you just ate. Accept that there will be days when you can't do the maximum. On those days, try to stick with the thirty minutes of accumulated moderate activity.

Remember: Your primary reason for exercise is to protect your health. Try to enjoy physical activity as an ongoing process in your life, not as a limited effort just to get in shape. Be adventurous. Try as many different activities as you can. You never know what may become your passion. Consider the time you may spend in aerobic exercise or strength training *your* time and try to lose yourself in the activity. Pace yourself and focus on how you feel, not on what the scale and the tape measure say. If you do set measurable goals, make them realistic and don't punish yourself if you fall short. Most important, remember that the real progress comes in learning to *enjoy* physical activity.

How to Find and Use a Personal Trainer

A personal trainer can help you design a safe, individualized plan for regular physical activity—and can help you stick to it. You can work with a trainer at a health club or in your own home. If you are thinking about hiring a trainer, here are some points to remember.

◆ Always check credentials and references. At a minimum, your trainer should have current certification from ACSM (American College of Sports Medicine, 317-637-9200), ACE (American Council on Exercise, 619-535-8227), NSCA (National Strength and Conditioning Association, 719-632-6722), or AFAA (Aerobics and Fitness Association of America, 800-446-2322). These organizations also can refer you to trainers in your area. Don't assume that all health club trainers are certified. Another good source for names of trainers is a local college physical education or exercise physiology department. Or, if you are already working with a nutrition professional, ask him or her for a recommendation.

◆ If possible, watch various trainers in action. Ask for a free sample workout before you make any long-term commitments. You and your trainer must be able to communicate well. See if he or she listens to you when you express your needs and goals. Make sure your trainer speaks to you in language you can understand—not scientific jargon.

◆ Make sure your trainer performs a fitness assessment before you begin serious work. Set short-term and long-term goals. Your trainer should reassess your fitness after about six weeks, and then every few months for as long as your sessions continue. Reassess your goals regularly, too. It will help keep you motivated.

◆ A basic program should include cardiovascular exercise (aerobic), strength training (weights) and flexibility (stretching). If your trainer wants you to do the cardiovascular work on your own, make sure he or she gives you a plan and keeps tabs on your progress.

◆ A good trainer should plan to make himself or herself obsolete—that is, to train you to take charge of your own plan. After several months of steady sessions, you should be able to reduce the time you spend with a trainer.

Choosing an Exercise Video

As you've probably realized, just about anyone can make an exercise video these days. Consequently, when you are purchasing one, you want it to be safe, effective and appropriate to your level of fitness. Here are some pointers.

◆ Match the video to your goals. If you're just getting started, skip the videos labeled "intermediate" or "advanced." Read the box to see if the program stresses aerobic activity, muscle strengthening, stretching or some combination of the three. If the video is a total body workout, the aerobics and strengthening segments should be at least twenty minutes each, not including warmup and cooldown.

◆ Make sure the instructor is certified by a recognized organization like ACSM, AFAA or ACE.

◆ Read as many video reviews as you can in various fitness magazines. Try to rent a tape or borrow it from the library or a friend before you commit to buying your own copy. The science of exercise changes over time, and outdated videos can range from ineffective to downright dangerous.

◆ Make your own tapes of television workout programs that often air early in the morning.

◆ Make sure you understand and can follow the instructor. He or she should motivate you and give you clear instructions. If the instructor's voice grates on your nerves or if he or she goes too fast, pick another tape. Getting frustrated and stressed out isn't the goal!

How to Choose a Health Club

All health clubs are not created equal. The International Association of Fitness Professionals suggests asking these questions to evaluate health clubs.

◆ Does the facility have adequate room and equipment—especially for peak hours? Are the temperature and air circulation comfortable?

◆ Does the facility have the cardiovascular equipment and weight-training equipment (free weights and machines) you want? Are there classes or programs you are interested in? Are they scheduled conveniently?

- Is the equipment clean and in good working condition? Are there signs/posters nearby that explain how to use equipment? Does the club hire qualified, certified trainers?
- Are there established health-emergency procedures and first-aid equipment? Does the club have liability insurance?
- Can you try out the facility free of charge before making a commitment to join? Are membership fees and policies clear?
- Is the facility close to home or work? Is it open at times that are convenient for you—early in the morning, for example?
- Are the employees friendly and eager to help you as an individual? Are you comfortable with the other members?

Benefits of Physical Activity by Life Stage

Age Group	Benefits
Children	- Helps build peak bone mass. - Establishes good, healthy lifestyle habits early in life. - Helps maintain a healthy weight. - Decreases likelihood of adult obesity. - Promotes heart health. - Prevents or delays development of high blood pressure.
Adolescents and young adult women	- Helps build peak bone mass. - May reduce risk of breast cancer. - Helps maintain a healthy weight. - Helps control body fat. - Promotes heart health. - Prevents or delays development of high blood pressure.

Premenopausal adult women	◆ Helps preserve existing bone.
	◆ May reduce risk of breast cancer.
	◆ Helps maintain a healthy weight.
	◆ Helps control body fat.
	◆ Promotes heart health.
	◆ May help reduce high blood pressure.
	◆ Helps prevent/treat diabetes.
Postmenopausal adult women	◆ Helps preserve existing bone and build new bone.
	◆ Enhances effect of hormone replacement therapy, calcium supplementation and osteoporosis drugs.
	◆ Helps maintain a healthy weight.
	◆ Helps control body fat.
	◆ Promotes heart health.
	◆ May help reduce high blood pressure.
	◆ Helps prevent/treat diabetes.
	◆ Helps fight depression.
Older women	◆ Slows decline in immune function.
	◆ Promotes strength, flexibility and coordination that lessen the likelihood of falling.
	◆ Helps preserve existing bone and builds new bone.
	◆ Enhances effect of hormone replacement therapy, calcium supplementation and osteoporosis drugs.
	◆ Helps prevent loss of muscle tissue.
	◆ Promotes heart health.
	◆ May help reduce high blood pressure.
	◆ Helps prevent/treat diabetes.

                                    ◆ Reduces arthritis pain.

    ◆ Improves sleep.

    ◆ May boost memory and mental alertness.

    ◆ Helps fight depression.

    ◆ May help body preserve needed protein.

Pregnant and lactating women (Always check with your physician before exercising vigorously.)

    ◆ Prevents excess weight gain; helps reduce discomforts of pregnancy.

    ◆ May increase volume of breast milk.

Points to Remember

For physical activity:

◆ **Anyone at any age can benefit from physical activity. In fact, the most dramatic health benefits occur when you make that first move from being a couch potato to becoming moderately fit.**

◆ **Try for thirty minutes of accumulated physical activity each day.**

◆ **Build bone and muscle with strength training. Boost your cardiovascular health with aerobic exercise. Enhance your flexibility with stretching.**

STRATEGY 3: REBALANCE YOUR DIET. ENJOY MORE FRUITS, VEGETABLES AND GRAINS AND LESS FAT

Some of the most exciting work being done in nutrition science today involves unlocking the health benefits of fruits, vegetables and grains. Naturally low in fat and high in carbohydrates, these foods are the best insurance against a host of diseases, and we're finding out more and more about them every day (see chapter 4).

I have put the emphasis on adding more fruit, vegetables and grains to your diet because it's not only a good way to get a lot of important nutrients, it's also a great way to cut down on fat. You just won't have enough room for a lot of high-fat food. In addition, the fiber in fruits, vegetables and grains helps lower cholesterol and keeps the digestive tract running smoothly. Some researchers believe fiber also plays a key role in preventing certain cancers. Antioxidants and phytochemicals in plant-based foods are thought to fight cancers, both by neutralizing damaging free radicals and by influencing the effects of estrogen. Fruits and vegetables are high in folic acid, a B vitamin that lowers blood levels of the heart-damaging amino acid homocysteine. And some recent research suggests that fruits and vegetables rich in potassium, magnesium, calcium, fiber and other nutrients may help lower blood pressure as effectively as drugs. (See chapter 4 for more on vitamins, minerals and phytochemicals.)

Yet despite the growing body of evidence supporting the benefits of a diet high in fruit, vegetables and grains, most of us fall short of the number of daily servings recommended in the Food Guide Pyramid—five servings a day of fruits and vegetables and six to eleven servings of grain (including three servings of whole grains). In fact, only one in five adults meets the fruit and vegetable guideline. For grains, the disparity is even greater. Most people are eating only about a half serving to one serving a day of whole grains, rather than the recommended three.

Retrain Your Taste Buds

◆ Switch to a lower-fat butter or margarine, then start using the product less frequently.
◆ Switch to leaner cuts of meat, then start reducing por-

tions and eating meat less frequently. Trim as much fat as you can from meat.

◆ Use less oil in cooking. Substitute fat-free broth, vegetable or fruit juice, Worcestershire sauce, flavored vinegar, wine or even water instead. Use nonstick cookware. When using oil, heat the skillet slightly before adding the oil. Warm oil will spread easily to coat the pan surface and you will use less. Foods also absorb less fat when the oil is warmed first.

◆ Use mustard on sandwiches instead of mayonnaise, or dilute mayonnaise with lemon juice, vinegar or tomato puree, so you will use less.

◆ Store cans of broth in the refrigerator. Fat will solidify on the surface, making it easy to remove.

◆ Skip the butter called for in packaged foods like rice and pasta mixes. You won't miss it.

◆ Blot the grease off the top of pizza with a napkin. You can eliminate as much as a teaspoon of fat—4.5 grams—per slice.

◆ Leave the last half inch or so of Asian takeout food in the container. You'll still get a taste of the sauce, but you'll avoid a lot of the fat.

◆ When ordering a side dish for eggs, remember that ham is leaner than bacon and bacon is leaner than sausage. (Ham is usually leaner than turkey sausage, too.)

◆ When buying ground turkey, make sure it's ground turkey *breast*. Regular ground turkey can include fatter darker meat and skin—making it equal to lean ground beef in fat content.

◆ Mash potatoes with skim milk and roasted garlic. Add a touch of olive oil if necessary.

◆ Thicken soup with pureed potato instead of milk or cream. You can also use mashed potato flakes, pureed beans, or roasted garlic, rice or cornstarch mixed with evaporated skim milk.

Substitutes

Instead of . . .	Use
1 whole egg	2 egg whites or 1/4 cup egg substitute
—in baking	mashed bananas or 2 tablespoons of cornstarch
—for binding	bread crumbs, tomato paste or oatmeal
Fudge sauce	chocolate syrup
Cocoa butter	powdered cocoa
Baking fats	prune puree, applesauce or canned pumpkin

How to Enjoy More Fruits, Vegetables and Grains

As you think about adding more plant-based foods to your diet, aim for balance and variety. Include a number of different types of foods—like whole grains, citrus fruits, green leafy vegetables, cruciferous vegetables, to name a few. Within each category, go for variety so you get the full benefit of all the nutrients these foods offer. For example, there is much more to citrus fruit than oranges and grapefruit. Don't stop at spinach and broaden your horizons beyond brown rice. Here are some tips for adding more fruits, vegetables and grains to your daily fare.

- Substitute vegetables for the meat in lasagna and other pasta recipes. Rich-tasting portobello mushrooms, for example, have a "meaty" texture. Add vegetables to marinara sauce.
- Double your normal serving size of vegetables.
- Grate a carrot into tuna salad.

◆ Keep a bowl of cut-up vegetables in plain view on the top shelf of the refrigerator.

◆ Add cooked lentils and beans to salads.

◆ Add chopped, firm tofu to salads, soups, stir-fries and pasta sauces.

◆ When you are in a hurry, use the salad bar at the grocery store for already cut-up fruits/vegetables.

◆ Start your day with two fruits—for example, orange, grapefruit or tomato juice and a sliced banana on cereal or toast.

◆ Make ice cubes of fruit juice and add them to sparkling water.

◆ Make frozen fruit kebobs with pineapple, bananas and strawberries.

◆ Add fruit to green salads and to chicken and tuna salads.

◆ Bake, stew or poach apples, pears or peaches with cinnamon, cloves and honey.

◆ Instead of jelly, add grated apple or chopped dates to a peanut-butter sandwich.

◆ Cook grains in fruit juice or vegetable juice instead of water.

◆ Add wheat germ to your cereal and to pancake and waffle mixes. Use it with ground turkey to make meat loaf or meatballs.

◆ Experiment with new grains. Quinoa, for example, is a good source of calcium. Use it instead of rice. Millet, which is high in B vitamins and iron, is good in stuffings and casseroles.

◆ Plan grains into every meal—for example, hot or cold cereal in the morning, whole-grain bread at lunch, brown rice or another grain at dinner.

When you are buying fresh produce, seasonal fruits and vegetables usually are your best choice—for nutrition, taste and cost. But don't dismiss frozen and canned fruits and vegetables. Nutritionally, they are often comparable to their fresh counterparts. Frozen spinach, canned peaches and apricots, and canned tomatoes are some examples.

Heat canned vegetables in their own liquid and use leftover liquid for soups and sauces. It usually contains significant nutrients. To avoid added sugar, look for canned fruits packed in fruit juice. Even then, it's a good idea to drain the fruit before using it.

Keeping an Eye on Fat

The second part of Strategy 3 involves lowering the fat in your diet. You probably know a lot about how to do this already. To test your fat IQ, take this quick quiz:

Do You Know Where the Fat Is?
True or False

1. Two percent milk is 98 percent fat free.   T or F
2. If heart health is your goal, you should
   eliminate red meat from your diet.   T or F
3. Regular (oil-roasted) nuts contain the same
   amount of fat as dry-roasted nuts.   T or F
4. "Lite" or reduced-calorie salad dressings
   always have less fat than regular dressings.   T or F
5. A skinned chicken thigh has more fat than
   a pork tenderloin.   T or F
6. A tablespoon of "lite" margarine has fewer
   calories than a tablespoon of sour cream.   T or F

Answers

1. False. The 2 percent refers to the weight of the fat in the milk, not the percentage of calories. Two percent milk actually has 38 percent calories from fat.
2. False. Lean beef and pork can be part of a low-fat diet. Choose "select" grades, eat moderate portions and use lean cooking methods like baking and broiling.

---

3. True. Because they are already high in fat, nuts don't absorb much fat when roasted in oil.
4. False. Some reduced-calorie salad dressings can be higher
   in fat than their full-calorie counterparts. Check the label.
5. True. The chicken has about twice the fat of the tenderloin, which is a particularly lean cut of pork.
6. False. A tablespoon of "lite" margarine has about six
   grams of fat; a tablespoon of sour cream has only about
   two grams of fat.

You can do some fairly simple things to keep your fat intake in
check without feeling deprived. Some researchers believe you can
retrain your taste buds away from a preference for fat (see sidebar
Retrain Your Taste Buds, page 198). But keep in mind that when
you try too hard to cut out the fat, you might cause more harm
than good. For example, some women avoid dairy products because they think foods like milk and cheese are fattening. But if you
drop the dairy from your diet, you're also eliminating the best
source of calcium and vitamin D (see Strategy 4). Remember: The
smart move isn't elimination; it's moderation. Switch to lower-fat
dairy products and use them wisely.

Figuring Out Fat

Calories per day	Recommended total fat grams per day (30% of calories)	Recommended total saturated fat grams per day (10% of calories)
1,600	53 or less	18 or less
2,000	65 or less	20 or less
2,200	73 or less	24 or less
2,500	80 or less	25 or less

Some women also banish red meat from their plates because it is high in saturated fat. The fact is you can enjoy small portions of lean red meat, which is a great source of protein and iron. Just think of meat more as a condiment or an accent to a meal rather than a main course. And if you do decide to eliminate all meat from your diet, balance your nutrient intake with a variety of legumes, which are good sources of protein.

In chapter 4, I explained in some detail why fat is an important nutrient. One reason is the great contribution it makes to flavor. As you "rebalance" your diet, don't underestimate the importance of taste. Just because you cut back on fat doesn't mean you have to cut back on flavor (see sidebar Boosting Low-Fat Flavor, page 205).

I believe it's also helpful to remember *why* you are trying to lower the amount of fat you eat. Think about it. We have been bombarded with low-fat messages for so long and have built up such guilt on the subject that many of us may have lost sight of exactly why we're buying all those fat-free foods and low-fat cookbooks.

The fact is that physicians and nutrition professionals recommend a diet low in fat for two basic reasons: to lower the risk for heart disease and to help maintain a healthy weight (which, in turn, lowers risks for a number of diseases such as diabetes, high blood pressure and some cancers).

Saturated fat in particular is implicated in heart disease because it raises blood cholesterol. *All* types of fat contribute to weight gain simply because they pack a lot of calories per gram. You can eat twice as much carbohydrate or protein compared to fat for about the same "price" in calories. If you stick to the number of calories you need to maintain a healthy weight but use up too many on high-fat food, you'll miss out on a lot of vital nutrients like the ones found in fruits, vegetables and grains.

We looked at the different types of fat in chapter 4 and reviewed the Dietary Guideline that recommends limiting total fat to 30

Boosting Low-Fat Flavor

Fat contributes so much to the pleasurable experience of food that we often miss it when it's gone. Here are some ideas for preserving flavor while cutting back on fat:

◆ Sprinkle flavored vinegar on sandwich bread or use roasted peppers instead of mayonnaise.

◆ Make your own salad dressing with small amounts of full-flavored oils like almond or sesame oil.

◆ Use sweetened fruit "butters," which actually don't contain any butter at all.

◆ Use high-quality, intensely flavored cheeses. Grate or shave just a little on salads, soups and pastas.

◆ Roast your vegetables. Roasting produces an intense flavor because it concentrates natural sugars. Use just a little olive oil (spray or brush it on), pepper and fresh or dried herbs.

◆ Puree chopped cantaloupe, add a dash of nutmeg and serve as a sauce over ice milk or low-fat frozen yogurt.

◆ Sprinkle jicama or cucumber spears with chili powder for a cool and zesty snack.

◆ Experiment with different types of bread to find flavors and textures that you don't want to mask with butter.

◆ When the taste of butter is essential, heat butter until it turns a light brown. Because the flavor from brown butter is stronger, you can use less.

◆ Experiment with fresh and dried herbs. In addition to adding flavor to food, herbs are also thought to offer some health benefits.

percent of calories and saturated fat to 10 percent of calories (see sidebar Figuring Out Fat, page 203). Of course, like all the Dietary Guidelines, the advice on fat is general because it must apply to the entire population—a very diverse group of people. You and your physician may decide, however, that you would benefit more from a diet somewhat high in monounsaturated fat, which could bring your total fat intake to over 30 percent of calories. Some experts believe that a diet in which only 20 percent of calories from fat— or even just 10 percent—might be the healthiest of all. Maybe so, but could many of us stick with it and enjoy it? Probably not.

I am convinced, however, that we can learn to enjoy a diet rich in carbohydrates—much more so than many of us do today. Try to make your food decisions mindfully, not mindlessly. When you make conscious decisions about the food you eat, you become more involved in the experience of eating and enjoy it more. Start by switching your focus from an obsession over fat to a passion for the taste and health benefits of fruit, vegetables and grains.

Benefits of a Diet High in Vegetables, Fruits and Grains and Low in Fat by Life Stage

Age	Benefits
Children	◆ Provides vitamins and minerals essential for growth.
(Fat intake of children under the age of two should not be restricted.)	◆ Establishes healthy eating habits.
	◆ Lowers risk of heart disease in later years.
	◆ Helps maintain a healthy weight.
	◆ May lower risk of breast cancer in later years.
Adolescents and young women	◆ Provides vitamins and minerals vital for growth.
	◆ Establishes healthy eating habits.

	◆ Lowers risk of heart disease in later years.
	◆ Helps maintain a healthy weight.
	◆ May lower risk of breast cancer in later years.
Premenopausal women	◆ Protects against breast cancer.
	◆ Helps maintain a healthy weight.
	◆ May lower risk of breast cancer.
	◆ Folic acid protects against birth defects.
	◆ Iron protects against anemia.
Postmenopausal women	◆ Helps maintain a healthy weight.
	◆ May lower risk of breast cancer.
	◆ Protects against heart disease.
	◆ Calcium supplements may be necessary.
Older women	◆ Helps maintain a healthy weight.
	◆ Protects against heart disease.
	◆ Fiber aids in digestion.
	◆ Calcium, magnesium and vitamin D supplements may be necessary.
Pregnant and lactating women	◆ Ensures mother and baby get all nutrients vital to growth and health.
	◆ Folic acid protects against birth defects.

Points to Remember

For rebalancing your diet:

◆ **Aim for five daily servings of fruits and vegetables plus six to eleven servings of grain, including three servings of whole grains.**

◆ **Enjoy a wide variety of fruits, vegetables and grains so you get some of all the nutrients they have to offer.**

- ◆ **The more fruits, vegetables and grains you eat, the less room you'll have for fat.**
- ◆ **Make your food choices a conscious decision.**

Tips

- ◆ Always check the labels of breakfast cereals. Some are fat free; others are higher in fat than you think.
- ◆ Watch your portion sizes. Low fat doesn't mean low calorie.
- ◆ To get your taste buds used to the sensation, try the low- or reduced-fat version of a product rather than going straight to the fat-free version. If you really like the low-fat version, stick with it.
- ◆ Healthy cooking equipment:
  Nonstick cookware
  Expandable stainless-steel or plastic steamer
  Gravy separator (for separating fats from pan juices)
  Pastry brushes (for applying a light coat of oil to pans and to vegetables for roasting)
- ◆ Practice the *art* of healthy eating: Choose the textured white, beige, pale yellow and honey brown of grains as your canvas (six to eleven servings/day). Add the vibrant red, yellow, orange, green and blue of vegetables rich in antioxidants and phytochemicals (five servings a day).

STRATEGY 4: GET ENOUGH CALCIUM

You might be wondering why I have singled out calcium for special attention. In any discussion about women's health and nutrition, calcium takes center stage because it is a major player in both the prevention and treatment of osteoporosis. A debilitating and costly bone disease, osteoporosis affects roughly twenty-five million Americans—most of them women. (See chapter 2.)

Almost all the calcium in your body can be found in your bones and teeth. And even though calcium is the most abundant mineral in your body, many things—like age, hormones, medications, other nutrients and even the time of day—can affect your ability to absorb calcium from food or supplements.

In addition to helping prevent osteoporosis, calcium also is vital to a number of basic body functions like regular heartbeat and blood clotting. And there is some evidence that calcium may help prevent hypertension as well as colon and breast cancer. Recent studies have also shown that calcium can be a marker for overall diet quality. If your diet is low in calcium, chances are good that it is low in a number of other key vitamins and minerals, too.

Calcium is such an important nutrient that, by law, calcium content must be listed on the nutrition panel of packaged foods. In fact, there is so much research showing the value of calcium that it is one of the few nutrients for which the government allows a health claim on food labels. In the next few years, you are likely to see a label statement on calcium-rich foods about calcium's role in preventing osteoporosis.

We have singled out calcium from among forty other nutrients not only because it plays such a critical role in maintaining good health, but also because women's lifestyles and their focus on being thin can interfere with getting enough calcium. It isn't found in large amounts in a lot of foods. In fact, dairy products alone contribute more than 75 percent of the calcium in our food supply. Yet many women, especially young women, think that all dairy foods are high in fat and avoid them for fear of weight gain. But if you eliminate milk, cheese and yogurt from your diet, you lose not only calcium, but also all the other vitamins and minerals dairy products offer.

Tips

◆ Drink three. Adult women need at least 1,000 mg of calcium a day: about the amount found in three glasses of milk.

◆ A sixteen-ounce latte (two shots of espresso in fourteen ounces of steamed milk) delivers 400 milligrams of calcium—40 percent of the average woman's daily needs. Order yours (or make your own) with skim milk.

◆ Add calcium-rich low-fat dried milk powder to recipes for soups and sauces.

◆ Dark green vegetables are good sources of calcium, but several servings are needed to equal the calcium found in just one glass of low-fat/skim milk. In addition, the calcium in dark greens is not absorbed as well as dairy calcium.

◆ To absorb calcium, you need about 400 international units of vitamin D each day, the amount found in four glasses of milk. In the South and Southwest, you can also get your vitamin D from year-round exposure to the sun—but be careful. Overexposure to the sun can cause skin cancer.

◆ Remember, a food does not have to be high in fat to be high in calcium.

◆ Spread your calcium intake throughout the day so your body can absorb it more easily.

◆ Loading up on calcium each day won't work. Your body has a threshold for calcium balance. After you reach that threshold, your body won't absorb any more.

What's in It for You?

As the population ages and life spans increase, osteoporosis is going to become even more prevalent in our society, especially for women. Research to identify early indicators of osteoporosis and better identify prevention techniques is ongoing. According to the National Institutes of Health, a woman who is fifty today has nearly one chance in two of developing osteoporosis in her remaining years. That's about five times the risk of developing breast cancer—which many surveys show is women's greatest health-related fear.

Women are especially vulnerable because they are generally smaller than men. We know that at menopause, women begin to lose bone as a result of lower levels of the hormone estrogen. Getting enough calcium is critical to help protect your bones at this time, especially if you choose not to take hormone replacement therapy. (For more about hormone replacement therapy, see chapter 3.)

As many as half of osteoporosis-related fractures could be prevented by a calcium-rich diet and regular exercise. Experts note that in osteoporosis prevention and treatment, calcium, exercise and estrogen are like the legs of a three-legged stool. It's hard to stay balanced without all three. In addition, recent research indicates that osteoporosis drugs like alendronate work even better when you are getting enough calcium.

Osteoporosis has no cure, but there are two means of prevention—and both rely on getting enough calcium. One is to increase what scientists call peak bone mass while you are young. Peak bone mass refers to the highest level of bone strength and density you are able to achieve. The other way to prevent osteoporosis is to slow down bone loss after menopause with calcium, exercise and, for some women, hormone replacement therapy and/or drugs.

Even though it may seem hard and unchanging, bone is actually dynamic, living tissue. When you are young and growing, calcium is "laid down" in your bones faster than it is removed. Adolescence is the very best time to build bones with lots of calcium-rich foods. And young girls retain significantly more calcium than women just a few years older. In middle age, as falling estrogen levels trigger changes in your body, a diet rich in calcium will help you protect the bone mass you have. After age sixty-five, you are likely to experience a sharp decline in calcium absorption.

Your physician may suggest that you have your bone density measured at menopause to establish a baseline against which to compare future bone loss. This test is a simple, painless X-ray procedure.

As a first step toward better managing the calcium in your diet, take this quiz.

---

*Do You Get Enough Calcium?**

Step 1. Take a minute to remember everything you ate yesterday at breakfast, lunch, dinner and for snacks.

Step 2. As you look at the chart of high-calcium foods below, write on the line next to each food how many servings you had yesterday. Make sure these are foods you usually eat. Put your number in the ☐ at the bottom of the high-calcium food chart.

    Combination Foods: Many things you eat contain a "combination" of foods. For example, a burrito may have tortillas, beans and cheese. Be sure to include servings in combination foods.

High-Calcium Foods

Milk and Milk Products	*Meats, Beans and Nuts*

*(1 cup milk, yogurt, pudding;
1 1/2 oz. cheese)*

__ nonfat or low-fat milk   __ sardines with bones
     or buttermilk   (6)
__ low-fat chocolate milk
__ nonfat or low-fat yogurt
__ low-fat cheese or mozzarella
     (1 1/2-in. cube)
__ whole milk
__ milk shake
__ hot chocolate
__ pudding
__ custard or flan
__ regular cheese (1 1/2-in. cube)

Number of High-Calcium Servings = ☐

Step 3. Look at the chart of medium-calcium foods below. Write on the line next to each food how many servings you had yesterday. Make sure these are foods you usually eat. Put your number in the ○ at the bottom of the medium-calcium food chart.

   Fortified Foods: Calcium is sometimes added to foods that don't contain it naturally—such as orange juice, cereal or bread. Check the nutrition label.

Medium-Calcium Foods

Milk and Milk Products (1/2 cup)	Meat, Beans and Nuts	Vegetables	Fruits	Breads, Cereals and Grains	Extras
_ nonfat or low-fat cottage cheese	_ dried beans or peas (1 cup)	_ bok choy (1 1/2 cups)	_ figs (5)	_ corn tortillas (2)	_ black strap molasses (1T)
_ cream soup	_ refried beans (1 cup)	_ broccoli (1 cup)			_ nonfat cream cheese (2T)
_ frozen yogurt	_ canned fish, with bones (salmon, mackerel) 2 oz.	_ kale (1 cup)			
_ ice milk	_ tofu processed with calcium (1/2 cup)	_ mustard greens (1 cup)			
	_ almonds (1/4 cup)	_ turnip greens (1/2 cup)			

Number of Medium-Calcium Servings = ○

Step 4. Using the guidelines that follow, convert your medium-calcium servings ○ to high-calcium equivalents and record your number in the ◇ below.

If your medium-calcium servings = ④ Count as 1 1/3 high-calcium servings

③ Count as 1 high-calcium serving

② Count as 2/3 high-calcium serving

① Count as 1/3 high-calcium serving

Your high-calcium equivalent number = ◇

Step 5. Add □ + ◇ to find your total calcium servings. Record your total here ▷

Step 6. Compare your total ▷ to the recommended number of calcium servings for your age group.

Number of Calcium Servings You Need Every Day

Preteens to Early 20s
1,200–1,500 milligrams ▷ 3–4 servings

Mid-20s to 30s and 40s
1,000 milligrams ▷ 2–3 servings

Pregnant or breast-feeding
1,200–1,500 milligrams ▷ 3–4 servings

From menopause on:
- ◆ Taking estrogen
  1,000 milligrams ▷ 2–3 servings
- ◆ Not taking estrogen
  1,500 milligrams ▷ 4 servings

*Reprinted by permission of Dairy Council of California

If you are like most women, you need to boost your daily calcium. The government's ongoing Nationwide Food Consumption study shows that after age eleven, no age group of females reaches even 75 percent of the amount of daily calcium now recommended by NIH. In fact, the average woman consumes only 300 to 500 milligrams of calcium a day—the equivalent of fewer than two cups of skim milk. That's only a third to a half of the 1,000 milligrams she needs.

Taking Charge of Your Calcium

Choose Food First: When making calcium choices, remember this simple guideline: Food, fortified food, supplements. The best way to get the calcium you need is to stick to foods *naturally* rich in calcium, such as milk. In fact, surveys have shown that if you don't eat dairy products, you will have a difficult time getting enough calcium. The next best way is to use calcium-fortified foods. Some brands of orange juice, breakfast bars, cereals and granola bars are fortified with calcium. Check the nutrition label for details. Product claims like "good source of calcium" and "rich in calcium" really mean something now. In the future, even more foods will have added calcium. Among items under consideration are potato chips, flour and rice.

Calcium supplements, though sometimes necessary, are the third choice for boosting your calcium intake. If you are post-menopausal, not taking HRT and don't eat at least four servings of food high in calcium (naturally or fortified), you should consider a

Lactose Intolerance Revisited

Some people, unable to digest lactose (the natural sugar in milk), experience bloating, abdominal cramps and flatulence when they drink milk. They are deficient in an enzyme called lactase, which breaks down lactose for digestion. Lactose-intolerant people do vary, however, in their ability to tolerate some milk products. New research shows that some lactose-intolerant individuals can tolerate up to one cup of milk a day.

A balanced diet should include two to three servings of low-fat dairy products each day. In addition to the many other nutrients milk products offer, they happen to be a primary source of calcium. If you suffer from some degree of lactose intolerance, try these strategies to help keep dairy foods in your diet.

- Drink smaller servings of milk (one-half cup). Consuming milk with meals can help reduce the symptoms of lactose intolerance. Try smaller servings of ice cream, yogurt and frozen yogurt, too.
- Choose naturally aged cheeses such as Swiss and Cheddar. They contain little or no lactose.
- Try yogurt with active cultures. The enzyme lactase is released by the bacterial cultures used to make yogurt and can temporarily substitute for the lactase your digestive system lacks.
- Experiment with lactose-reduced dairy products, enzyme preparations designed to reduce lactose and lactase tablets.

supplement. Some physicians and nutritionists recommend that all women, regardless of their circumstances, boost a calcium-rich diet with a supplement. This is a personal matter you should discuss thoroughly with your physician so that you always make a fully informed choice. Remember that relying on calcium supplements alone means you'll miss out on all the other important nutrients in calcium-containing foods.

Calcium carbonate, the form of calcium found in antacid tablets like Tums and Rolaids, is the most common supplement. It is economical and contains the highest concentration of calcium (elemental calcium) by weight. Take doses of 500 milligrams or less between meals to ensure that other nutrients don't interfere with absorption. Take your last supplement at bedtime; bone loss is thought to accelerate at night.

Some women, especially older women, may not have enough gastric acid in their stomachs between meals to absorb calcium carbonate effectively. If your physician determines that you fall into this category, you may want to take calcium carbonate with food so that the acid produced during digestion can help with absorption. Another alternative is to take calcium citrate. This form has less elemental calcium (so you'll need to take more of it) but does not need gastric acid for absorption.

The National Osteoporosis Foundation recommends sticking with brand-name supplements. Always check the label for the designation "USP" from the U.S. Pharmacopoeia. It means the supplement has been proven to dissolve well.

What's in It for You

Calcium Type	Percent Elemental Calcium	Elemental Calcium in 500-Milligram Tablet
Calcium carbonate	40	200 milligrams
Calcium citrate	21	105 milligrams

Learn Label Lingo: Food labels will help you make healthy food selections. Check the label for three types of information:

Nutrition Facts

Serving Size 1 cup (248g)
Servings Per Container 4

Amount Per Serving

Calories 150   Calories from Fat 35

	% Daily Value*
Total Fat 4g	**6%**
Saturated Fat 2.5g	**12%**
Cholesterol 20mg	**7%**
Sodium 170mg	**7%**
Total Carbohydrate 17g	**6%**
Dietary Fiber 0g	**0%**
Sugars 17g	
Protein 13g	

Vitamin A 4%	•	Vitamin C 6%	
Calcium 40%	•	Iron 0%	

* Percent Daily Values are based on a 2,000 calorie diet. Your daily values may be higher or lower depending on your calorie needs:

		Calories:	2,000	2,500
Total Fat	Less than		65g	80g
Sat Fat	Less than		20g	25g
Cholesterol	Less than		300mg	300mg
Sodium	Less than		2,400mg	2,400mg
Total Carbohydrate			300g	375g
Dietary Fiber			25g	30g

◆ **Nutrition panel:** Listing calcium content on the nutrition label is mandatory.

◆ **Label claim:** A product may also make label claims such as "high in calcium" or "good source of calcium." Claims like this should lead you to the nutrition label, where you can find out exactly how much calcium is in a serving.

◆ **Health claim:** The government allows health claims in seven areas related to disease prevention. A food manufacturer can put language on a label about calcium helping to lower risk for osteoporosis if that product meets some very strict criteria on calcium content.

Move Right Along: Regular physical activity is important not only for heart health but also for bone health. Exercise and nutrition go hand in hand. Researchers strongly suspect that regular weight-bearing exercise is especially important in calcium retention and in building bones. See the chart below to find some weight-bearing activities that you can enjoy on a daily basis, and work them into your overall program.

Weight-Bearing Exercise	*Non-Weight-Bearing Exercise*
Walking, hiking, jogging, running	Swimming
Tennis	Bicycling
Skiing	Stretching
Skating	Yoga
Weight lifting	

Use It. Don't Lose It: Other nutrients can affect your ability to use calcium. Consequently, even though you may be eating calcium-rich foods, your body may not be able to absorb all the calcium you need. But if you follow a well-balanced diet that includes a variety of foods in moderation, chances are you will not only get all the nutrients you need but also keep those nutrients working in harmony.

Keeping Calcium Wasters in Check

◆ Carbonated drinks contain as much as 75 milligrams of phosphorous per twelve ounces. Keep your daily intake to a maximum of 800 to 1,000 milligrams, or in a 1:1 ratio with your calcium intake.

◆ A diet too high in protein can result in loss of calcium through the urine. Forty to 80 grams of protein a day is the recommended level.

◆ Keep your daily sodium intake to a maximum of 2,000 to 4,000 milligrams per day. Too much sodium can cause loss of calcium through the urine.

Here are some of the nutrients that can affect calcium absorption (see also chapter 4):

◆ Vitamin D enhances calcium absorption. But as you age, your risk for vitamin D deficiency increases because your body doesn't absorb it as well. Sunlight as well as vitamin D–fortified milk and dairy products are the best source of this nutrient.

◆ If you eat a lot of salt or sodium-rich foods, you may increase calcium loss through your urine. For every 2,300 milligrams of sodium you eat, you lose 40 to 80 milligrams of urinary calcium. But that's not the only reason to moderate your sodium intake. A high-sodium diet can aggravate high blood pressure, too. One teaspoon of salt contains about 2,000 milligrams of sodium. Although health experts recommend limiting sodium to 2,400 milligrams per day, the typical American consumes about 4,000 to 5,000 milligrams of sodium daily, much of it in processed foods. Check the nutrition panel for sodium content.

◆ Too much protein can also affect your calcium retention. For every gram of protein you eat, your urinary calcium increases by about one milligram. Check with your registered dietitian to be sure the amount of protein you usually eat each day is in balance with other nutrients in your diet. For example, in a 2,000-calorie-a-day diet, experts recommend fifty grams of protein. The Food Guide Pyramid (see chapter 4) recommends two to three daily servings of meat, fish or poultry. Dairy products are also a good source of protein.

◆ Some foods, when eaten in excess, can interfere with calcium absorption. They include spinach (oxalates), wheat bran, and colas and processed foods (phosphorous). You don't need to eliminate these foods from your diet, but they should be eaten in moderation—especially colas and processed foods, which can contain extra sugar, salt and fat.

◆ Not only can other nutrients interfere with calcium absorption, but calcium itself can interfere with how your body uses other nutrients such as phosphorous, magnesium and iron. These minerals are plentiful in the food supply, so if you are eating a balanced diet, you should have no problem.

◆ The following medications may interfere with calcium absorption: steroids, thyroid hormones, aluminum-containing antacids, some anticonvulsants, lithium, some antibiotics and some anticancer drugs. If you are on any of these medications, check with your registered dietitian about taking a calcium supplement, perhaps one fortified with vitamin D.

Sources of Vitamin D

Sunlight
Vitamin D–fortified milk and cereal
Cod-liver oil
Fatty fish

Pass It Up. Pass It Down: Many women mistakenly think that getting enough calcium is important only at menopause. The truth is that osteoporosis prevention is a lifelong process, requiring what health experts call an "intergenerational" effort. If you have an adolescent or young-adult daughter or granddaughter, encourage her to eat calcium-rich foods. These early years are a window of opportunity for building the bone density that will be so important in her future. If you have a loved one approaching or going through menopause, encourage her to balance the bone loss caused by decreasing estrogen with adequate calcium. And for the older women in your life, encourage calcium and vitamin D–rich foods along with exercise to preserve bone health.

Daily Calcium Needs by Life Stage
National Institutes of Health
Infants

Birth–6 months	400 mg	◆ Is critical to growth and bone development.
6 months–1 year	600 mg	◆ Calcium absorption in exclusively breast-fed babies is significantly higher than in infants fed a cow-milk-based formula. To compensate for this discrepancy, formula makers boost the calcium in their products to nearly twice the content of human milk.
		◆ Low-birth-weight babies may need even more daily calcium than the recommended amount.

Children

1–5 years	800 mg	◆ Helps build peak bone mass.
6–10 years	800– 1,200 mg	◆ Prevents tooth decay.
		◆ During the first year of life, bones grow rapidly. Children retain less calcium than infants do, and they need two to four times as much calcium as adults do.
		◆ Studies have shown that a daily calcium intake of more than 800 mg may help children in the 6-to-10-year-old category increase their rate of bone accumulation.

Adolescents and young adults

| 11–24 years | 1,200– 1,500 mg | ◆ Helps build peak bone mass and achieve genetically determined height. |

◆ Calcium absorption during the preteen years is very efficient. During a teen girl's growth spurt (between 11 and 15 years of age), she will reach about 20 percent of her adult height.

Adult women

25–50 years Over 50 years (postmenopausal)	1,000 mg	◆ Helps build bone mass into the 30s.
—On estrogen	1,000 mg	◆ Helps protect bones after estrogen loss at menopause.
—Not on estrogen	1,500 mg	◆ In combination with estrogen and exercise, can help build new bone after menopause. ◆ Boosts the action of osteoporosis drugs.

Older adult women

Over 65 years	1,500 mg	◆ Helps reduce risk of osteoporosis-related fracture. ◆ May need supplemental vitamin D for optimal calcium absorption.

Pregnant and lactating women

	1,200– 1,500 mg	◆ Prevents permanent decline in mother's body calcium during pregnancy and lactation. ◆ Bone loss during lactation is rapidly restored after weaning. ◆ Reduces risk for pregnancy-induced hypertension and pre-eclampsia.

Points to Remember

Concerning calcium in your diet:

◆ Calcium is an important nutrient for women of *all* ages.
◆ If your diet is low in calcium, chances are it is low in other key nutrients, too.
◆ Calcium works best in preventing bone loss and building new bone when it is teamed up with exercise and estrogen.

Epilogue

I hope our shared journey has left you invigorated by new ideas and renewed in your sense of personal power. You will travel forward from here on your own—in your own time and in your own way.

It is true that as a woman you are particularly vulnerable to certain diseases. And, yes, there are certain risk factors you can't change. But you can control what you eat, and the evidence is mounting daily that nutrition has a profound effect on health throughout your life. No matter what your age, *now* is the time to take charge of your nutritional health. I urge you to use this book—and the principles of balance, variety and moderation on which it is based—as a framework to guide your everyday eating and exercise decisions.

I hope you also will remember that although each of us has our unique needs, we are part of the whole of women's health. As the gradual changes you make create a new and healthier way of life, you will have the opportunity to influence other women, both friends and family, young and old. This intergenerational sharing is not only a gift to your loved ones; it also creates the awareness and grassroots momentum necessary to keep women's nutrition and health high on the national agenda.

And as you follow your own path, you can continue the work of the dedicated advocates who cleared the way for you by demanding excellence from your health-care providers, by supporting women's health research and by using your vote to influence how health policy at every level of government is created and implemented.

The old saying is still true: A woman's work is never done. But I hope you agree that taking charge of your nutritional health is one job you can't afford to decline.

Resources

General

The American Dietetic Association
National Center for Nutrition and Dietetics
Consumer Nutrition Hot Line
800-366-1655
900-225-5267

National Health Information Center
U.S. Department of Health and Human Services
800-336-4797

Breast Cancer

American Cancer Society
800-ACS-2345

Cancer Care Hot Line
800-813-HOPE

Federal Cancer Information Center
800-4-CANCER

National Alliance of Breast Cancer Organizations
212-719-0154

National Cancer Institute
800-422-6237

National Coalition for Cancer Survivorship
301-650-8868

National Society of Genetic Counselors
610-872-7608

Susan G. Komen Breast Cancer Foundation
800-462-9273

Y-Me
800-221-2141

Diabetes

American Association of Diabetes Educators
800-832-6874

American Diabetes Association
800-232-3472

International Diabetes Center
612-993-3393

National Diabetes Information Clearinghouse
301-654-3327

National Institute of Diabetes and Digestive and Kidney Diseases
Prevention Study
888-377-5646

Heart Disease

American Heart Association
800-242-8721

National Heart, Lung and Blood Institute
301-496-4236

Office on Smoking and Health
Center for Chronic Disease Prevention and Health Promotion
707-488-5705

Obesity

Weight Control Information Network (WIN)
800-946-8098

Osteoporosis

National Dairy Council
800-426-8271

National Fluid Milk Promotion
Board "Milk, Where's Your Mustache?" Campaign
800-WHY-MILK (800-949-6455)

National Osteoporosis Foundation
202-223-2226

For a bone density testing location near you:
800-464-6700

Index

About the Author

Susan Calvert Finn, Ph.D., R.D., F.A.D.A., is a former president of The American Dietetic Association. As one of the country's leading nutrition and health communicators, she is a chief architect of ADA's Nutrition and Health Campaign for Women, and continues to spearhead the effort, serving as its primary spokesperson. Susan Finn is one of a prestigious group of health care leaders who recently convened at the National Institutes of Health's "Women's Health Strategies for the 21st Century." She is currently Director of Nutrition and Health Care Services, responsible for education, marketing, and government programs at Ross Products Division of Abbott Laboratories in Columbus, and holds a clinical professorship in the College of Medicine at The Ohio State University.